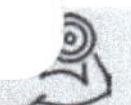

WORKOUT 3

2 A EZ-BAR BICEPS CURL

SETS 4 REPS 10 TEMPO 2010 REST 10sec

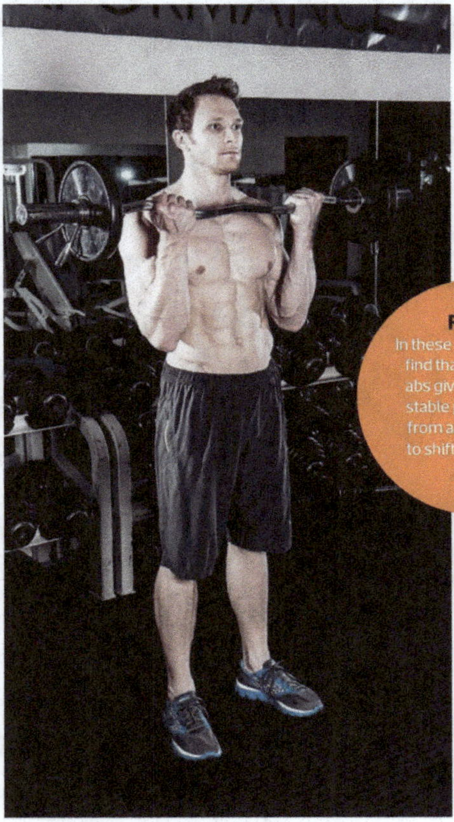

2 B EZ-BAR TRICEPS EXTENSION

SETS 4 REPS 10 TEMPO 2010 REST 45sec

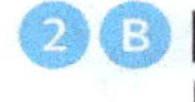

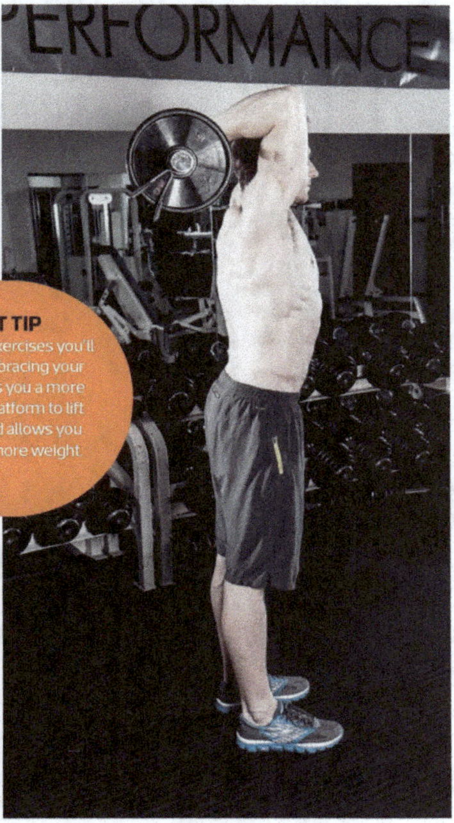

FIT TIP
In these exercises you'll find that bracing your abs gives you a more stable platform to lift from and allows you to shift more weight

Using an EZ-bar reduces stress on your elbows. Stand straight and curl the bar upwards. Squeeze your biceps at the top of the movement and your triceps at the bottom.

Stand holding an EZ-bar above your head, palms facing behind you. Lower the bar behind your head by bending your elbows. Pause, and then lift the weight by contracting your triceps.

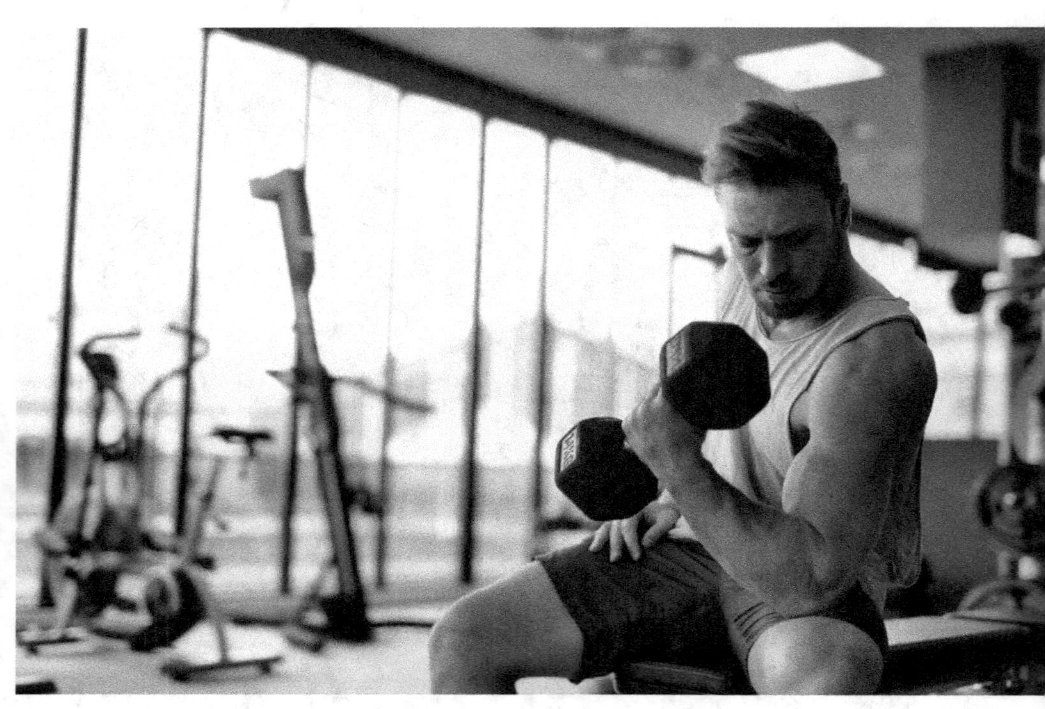

**MUSCLE
AFTER
40
Dominique rusch**

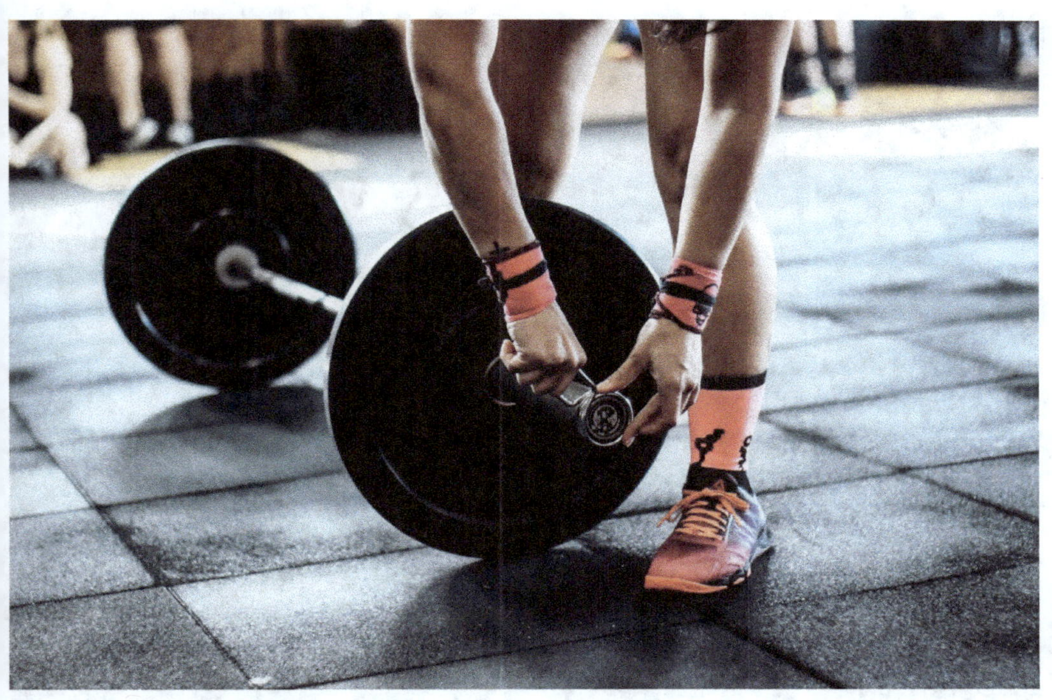

GET FIT FOR
LIFE

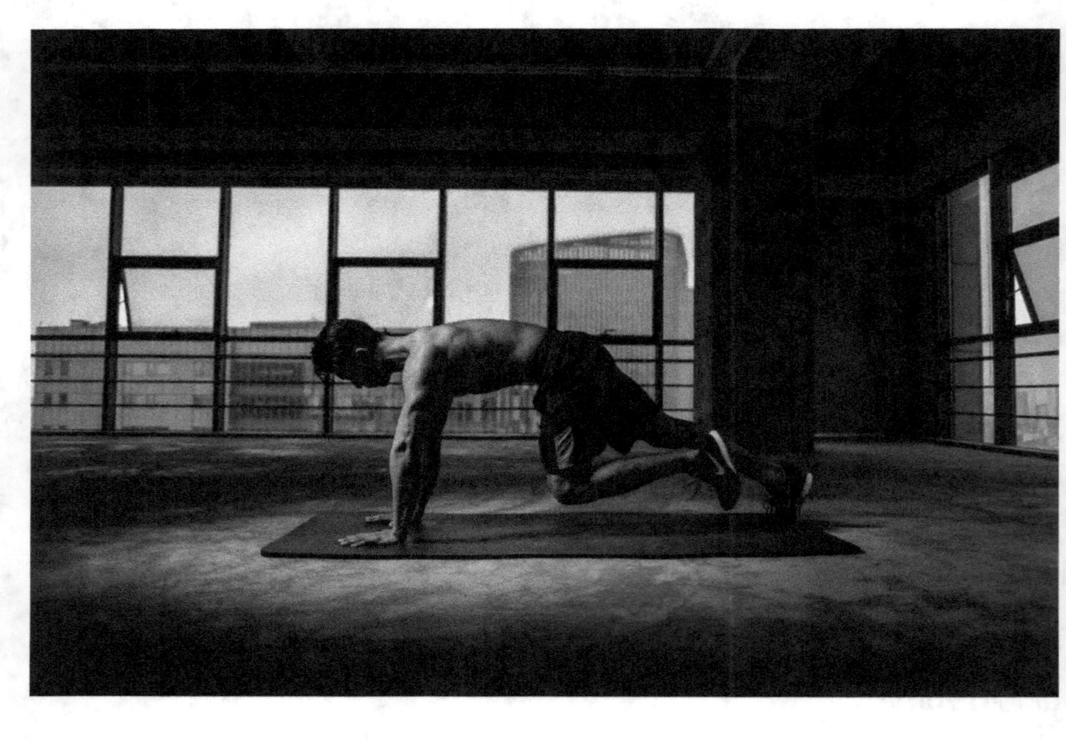

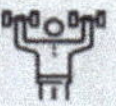

CONTENTS

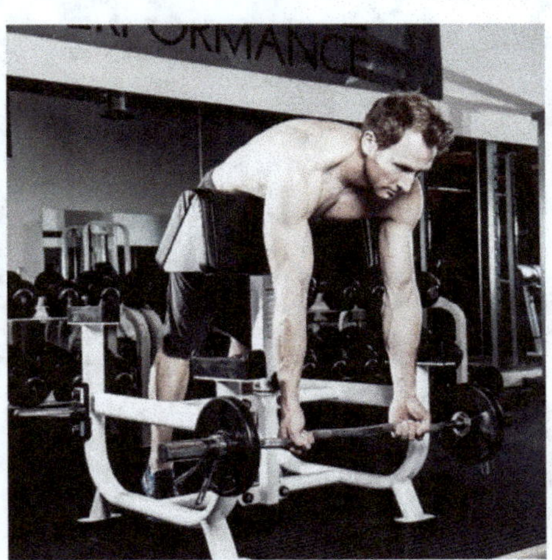

PHASE 2
STRENGTH

Introduction	**p52**
Week 1 Workout 1	**p56**
Week 1 Workout 2	**p60**
Week 1 Workout 3	**p64**
Week 1 Workout 4	**p68**
Week 2	**p72**
Week 3 Workout 1	**p74**
Week 3 Workout 2	**p78**
Week 3 Workout 3	**p82**
Week 3 Workout 4	**p86**
Week 4	**p90**

PHASE 1
FOUNDATIONS

Introduction	**p12**
Week 1 Workout 1	**p16**
Week 1 Workout 2	**p20**
Week 1 Workout 3	**p24**
Week 1 Workout 4	**p28**
Week 2	**p32**
Week 3 Workout 1	**p34**
Week 3 Workout 2	**p38**
Week 3 Workout 3	**p42**
Week 3 Workout 4	**p46**
Week 4	**p50**

PHASE 3
HYPERTROPHY

Introduction	**p92**
Week 1 Workout 1	**p96**
Week 1 Workout 2	**p100**
Week 1 Workout 3	**p104**
Week 1 Workout 4	**p108**
Week 2	**p112**
Week 3 Workout 1	**p114**
Week 3 Workout 2	**p118**
Week 3 Strenkout 3	**p122**
Week 3 Workout 4	**p126**
Week 4	**p130**

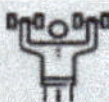

WELCOME!

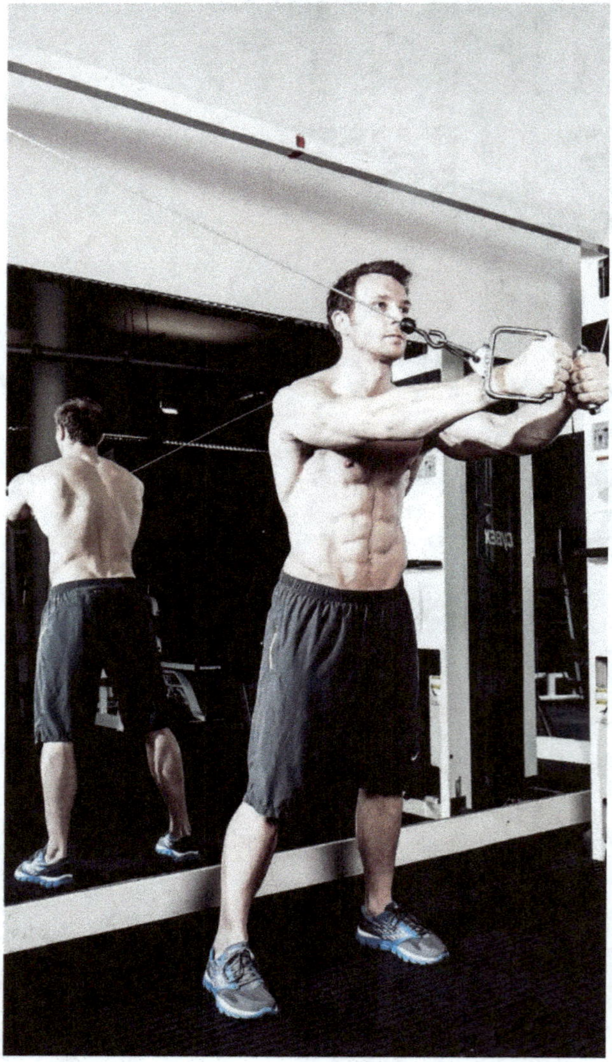

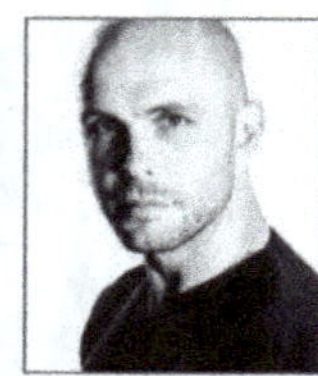

Building muscle after 40 might seem more challenging, but it's absolutely achievable with the right approach and mindset. One universal truth in both fitness and life is that we often overestimate what can be done in a week, yet underestimate what can be accomplished in three months. I've witnessed it countless times: if you've waited until just before a big event to start building muscle, even the most ambitious plan can't deliver instant results. However, if your target date is 12 weeks away, you're in the perfect position to transform your physique, and this guide will help you get there.

We have harnessed nearly two decades of expertise in muscle-building specifically tailored for those over 40, to create a programme that helps you get stronger and healthier swiftly while respecting your body's unique needs. Commit now, as you read this, to engage fully with this programme – both in the gym and in your daily routine – and you'll be amazed at what you can achieve. What happens in the three months beyond is up to you, but it all starts here.

Joel Snape Editor
@JoelSnape

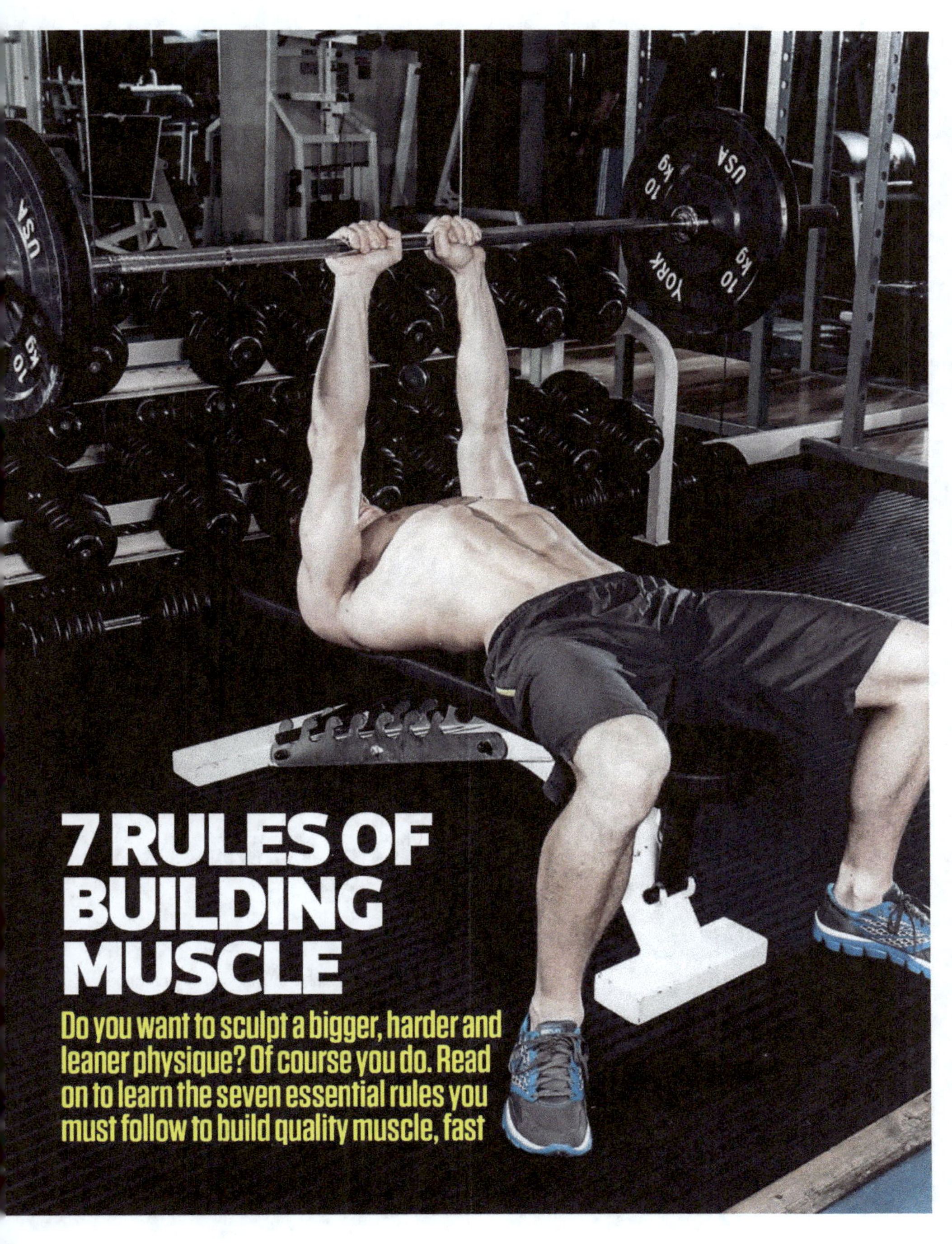

7 RULES OF BUILDING MUSCLE

Do you want to sculpt a bigger, harder and leaner physique? Of course you do. Read on to learn the seven essential rules you must follow to build quality muscle, fast

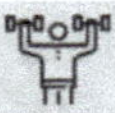

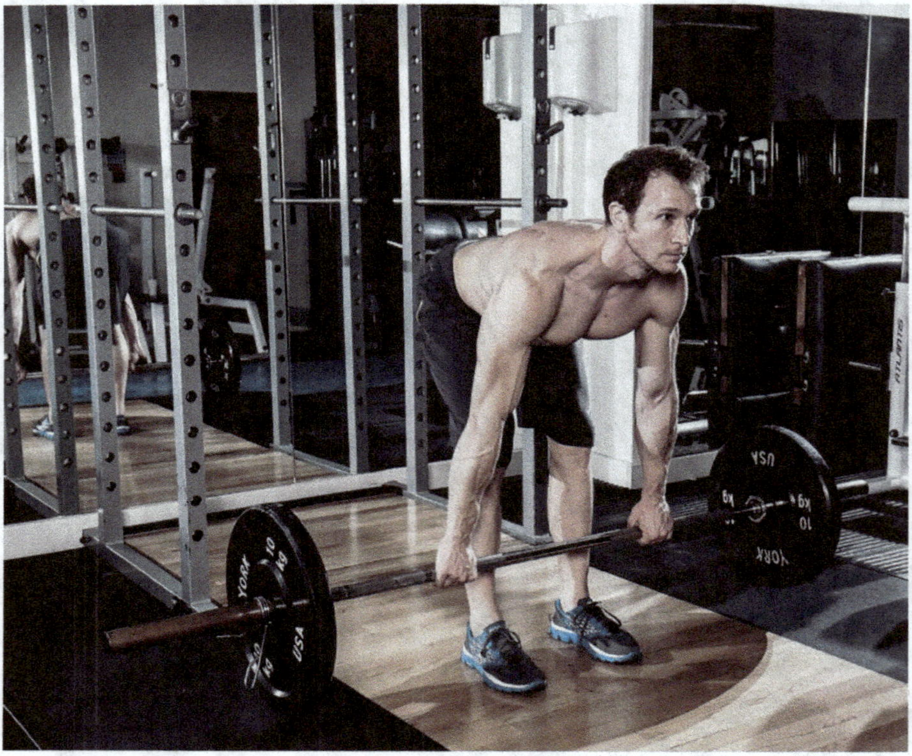

RULE 1
HAVE A PLAN

Walk into the gym without knowing exactly what you want to achieve and you're going to end up training at random. Not ideal for results. You've made a start on this rule simply by picking up this book, but take it further by making a back-up plan in case your preferred kit isn't available: that way, if someone's curling in the squat rack, you won't be stymied for long.

RULE 2
KNOW YOUR MOVES

Before you even think about picking up a dumbbell or loading up a barbell, you need to understand how to perform all the exercises that make up your workout. This is crucial not only to prevent injury, but also to ensure that every rep of every lift hits the target muscle or muscles effectively so you get better results in less time. Even if you think you know how to do the moves in this book, take time to check the form guides.

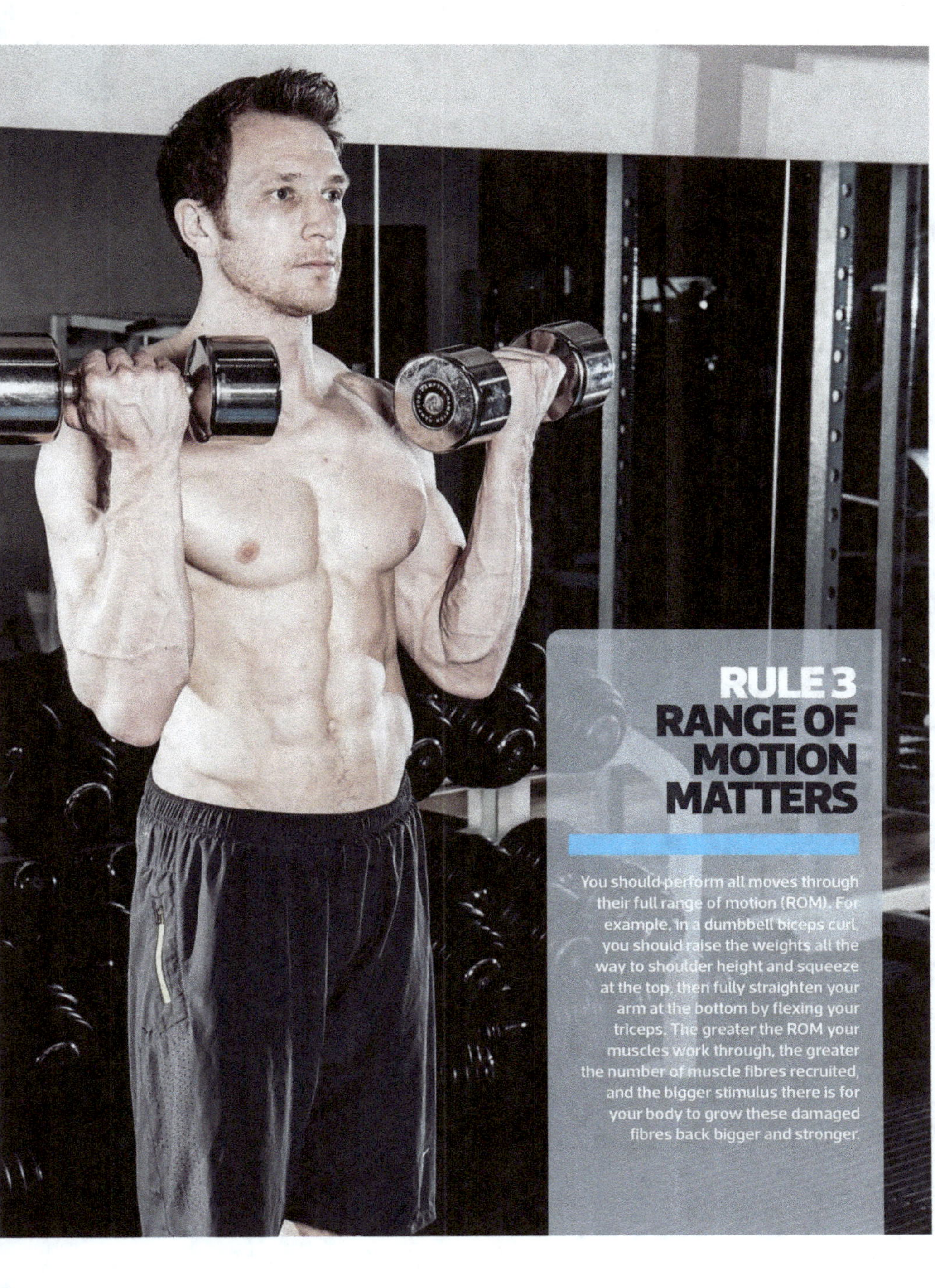

RULE 3
RANGE OF
MOTION
MATTERS

You should perform all moves through their full range of motion (ROM). For example, in a dumbbell biceps curl, you should raise the weights all the way to shoulder height and squeeze at the top, then fully straighten your arm at the bottom by flexing your triceps. The greater the ROM your muscles work through, the greater the number of muscle fibres recruited, and the bigger stimulus there is for your body to grow these damaged fibres back bigger and stronger.

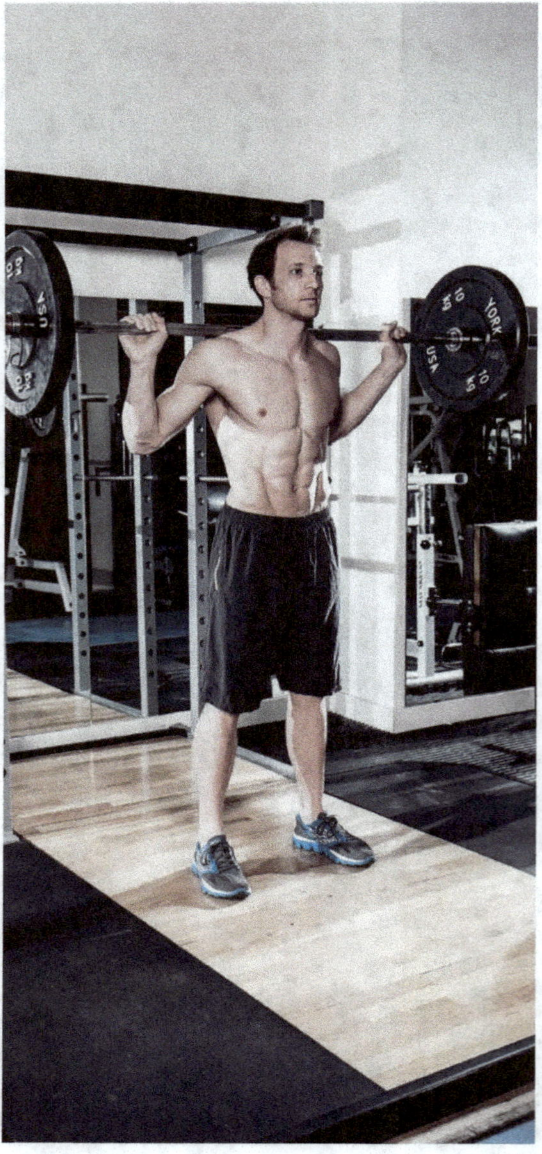

RULE 4
CHOOSE THE RIGHT WEIGHT

How do you know you have chosen the right weight? The final couple of reps of the first few sets should feel hard, and the final reps of the final sets should be very challenging. If you finish all the reps and feel like you could have done another five, the weight is too light; if you can only perform half the target number of reps before your muscles fail, the weight is too heavy. Selecting your starting weight for each exercise may require a little trial and error. If in doubt it's best to start light, then increase the weight in subsequent sets – or even do an extra set – instead of starting too heavy and not being able to finish the set.

RULE 5
INCREASE TIME UNDER TENSION

When it comes to hypertrophy (muscle growth), the weight, sets and reps you use are arguably less important than the time your muscles spend under tension (TUT). This is what will force them to grow. This plan uses tempo recommendations to control your TUT – by lifting a weight for two seconds and lowering it for four, you might make a single set last for 60-90 seconds, rather than the 15-30 it would take if you did it without considering tempo. The result? More muscular damage – and faster growth.

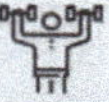

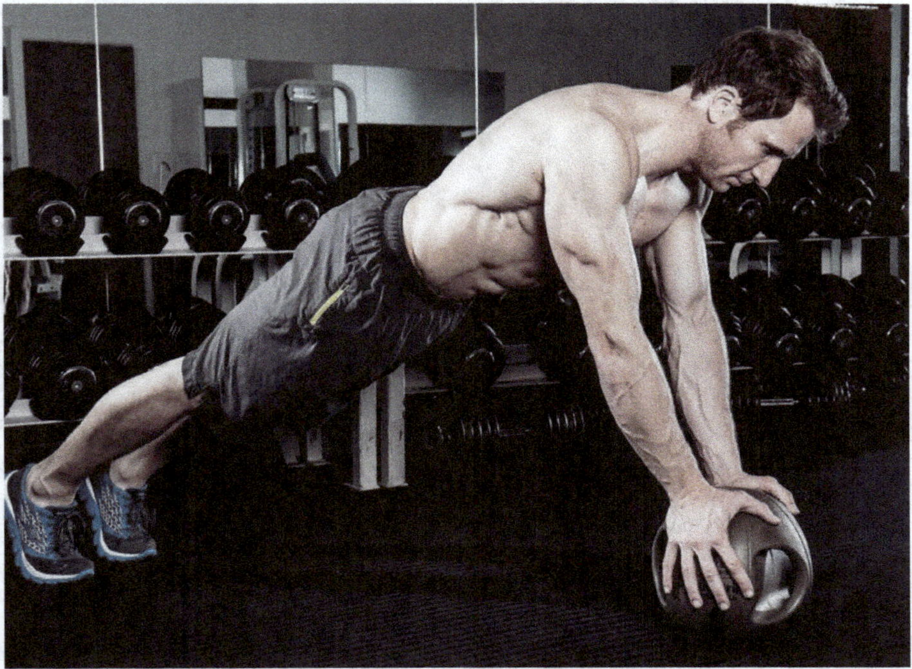

RULE 6
USE YOUR MIND

Forging better mind-to-muscle connections will go a long way towards building new muscle mass faster. All this means is that when you are performing each rep, you focus on the muscles that are working to move the weight: for instance, making sure your pecs are activating throughout a bench press, rather than letting your triceps take over. Literally looking at the muscle, either directly or in a mirror, is a great way to connect your mind to that muscle and make it work as hard as possible. Simply slinging a weight around won't give you the results you want.

RULE 7
EXECUTE WITH INTENT

You need to start every single session with the mentality that this is going to be the best workout you've ever had. Attacking each set with a sense of intent, purpose and positivity goes a long way to getting out of your comfort zone, which is where you need to be if you want to make big changes to your body fast. Shut out thoughts about problems at work, an argument with the missus or the want-away striker whose departure will ruin next season. Instead, put your phone on airplane mode, stick on your headphones, turn up the volume and lift like your life depends on it.

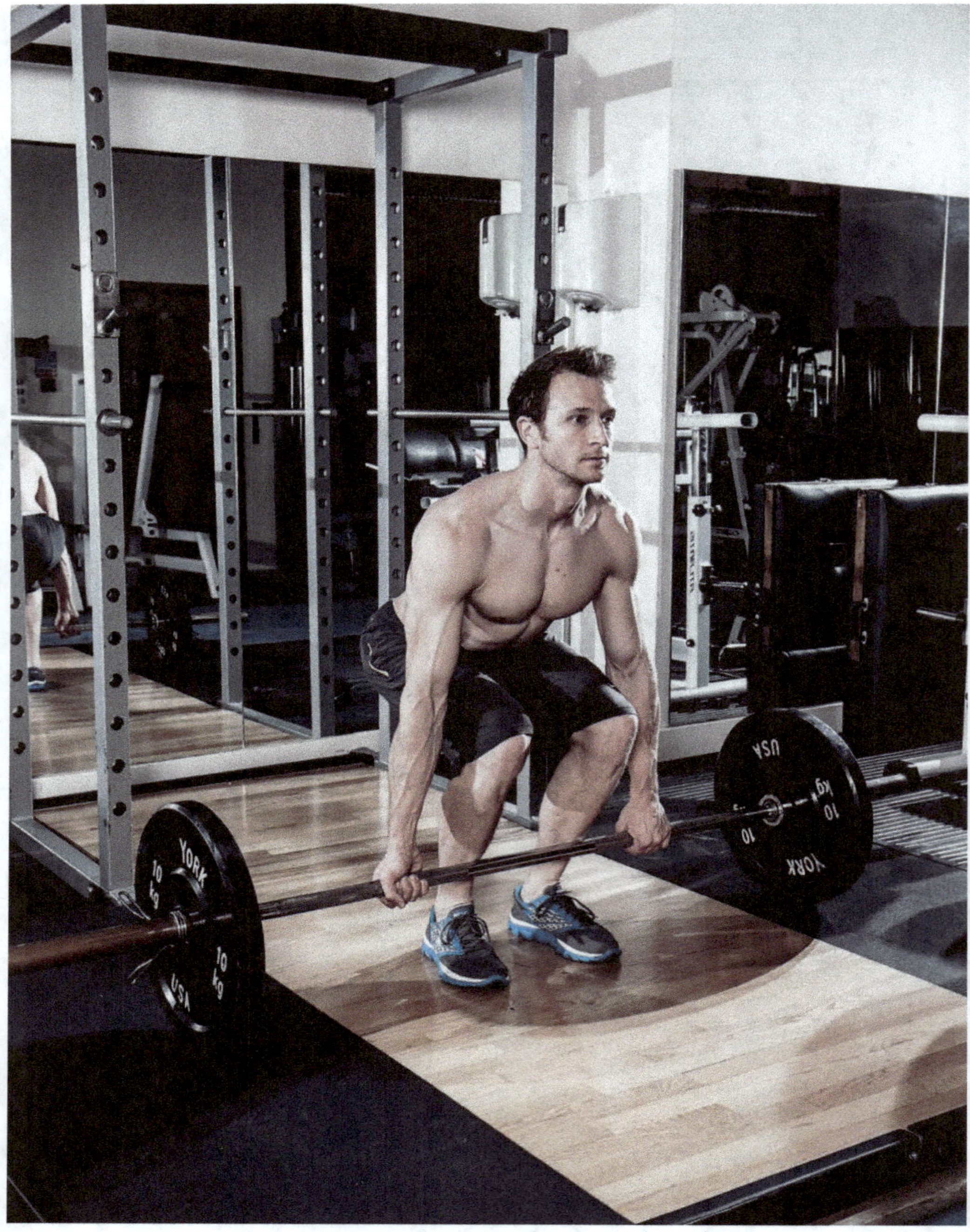

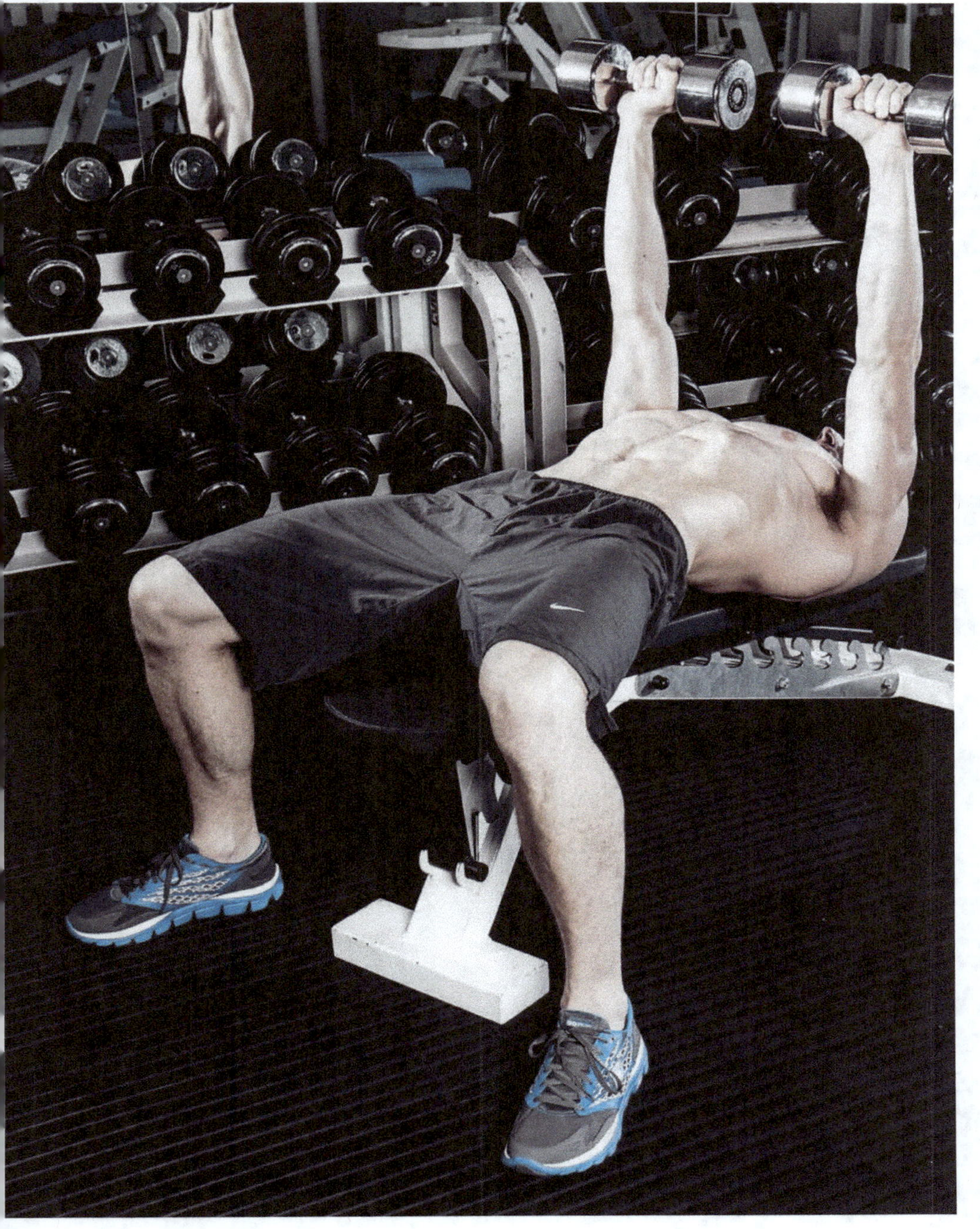

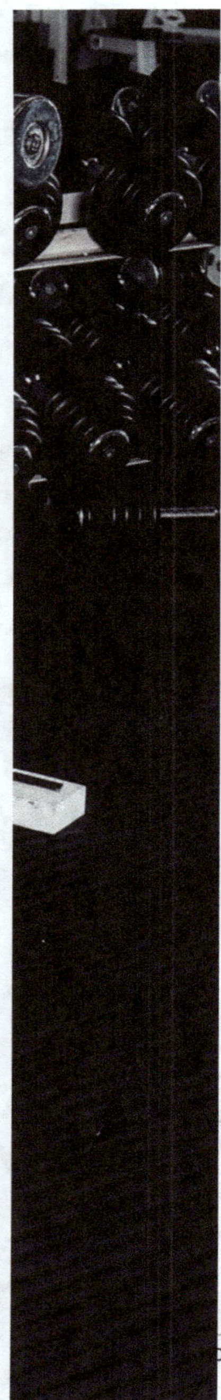

BUILD YOUR FOUNDATIONS

Over the first four weeks of the plan, you'll master the big dumbbell and barbell lifts, setting the stage for big gains later

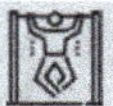

TRAIN SMARTER – AND HARDER

The aim of the first four-week phase of your training is simple: build firm foundations so that everything else is easier. If you've never lifted before, this is where you'll familiarise yourself with the movements that form the rest of the plan, focusing on one move at a time and taking generous rests so that you can nail every set.

Even if you're a gym veteran, it's worth doing: consider this phase a reset, a time to reassess your approach to the moves, focusing on form and tempo to make them more effective. The bench press is a classic example – sure, you can bang out a handful of sloppy reps, but make them slow, controlled and think about activating your pecs as you do them, and you'll build a mind-muscle connection that will give you huge benefits in the weeks to come.

In this phase, you split your training into upper-body and lower-body workouts, doing two of each every week. For beginner and intermediate lifters this is absolutely the best way to train, since you simply can't bring the same focus and intensity to, say, an arms-only session that requires a full week of rest before the next one. With this method, you'll combine pushing and pulling movements that tax your body to the limit, then get a couple of days' rest before you work on the same body parts again. Build your foundations well, and you'll be stronger and bigger in 12 weeks' time.

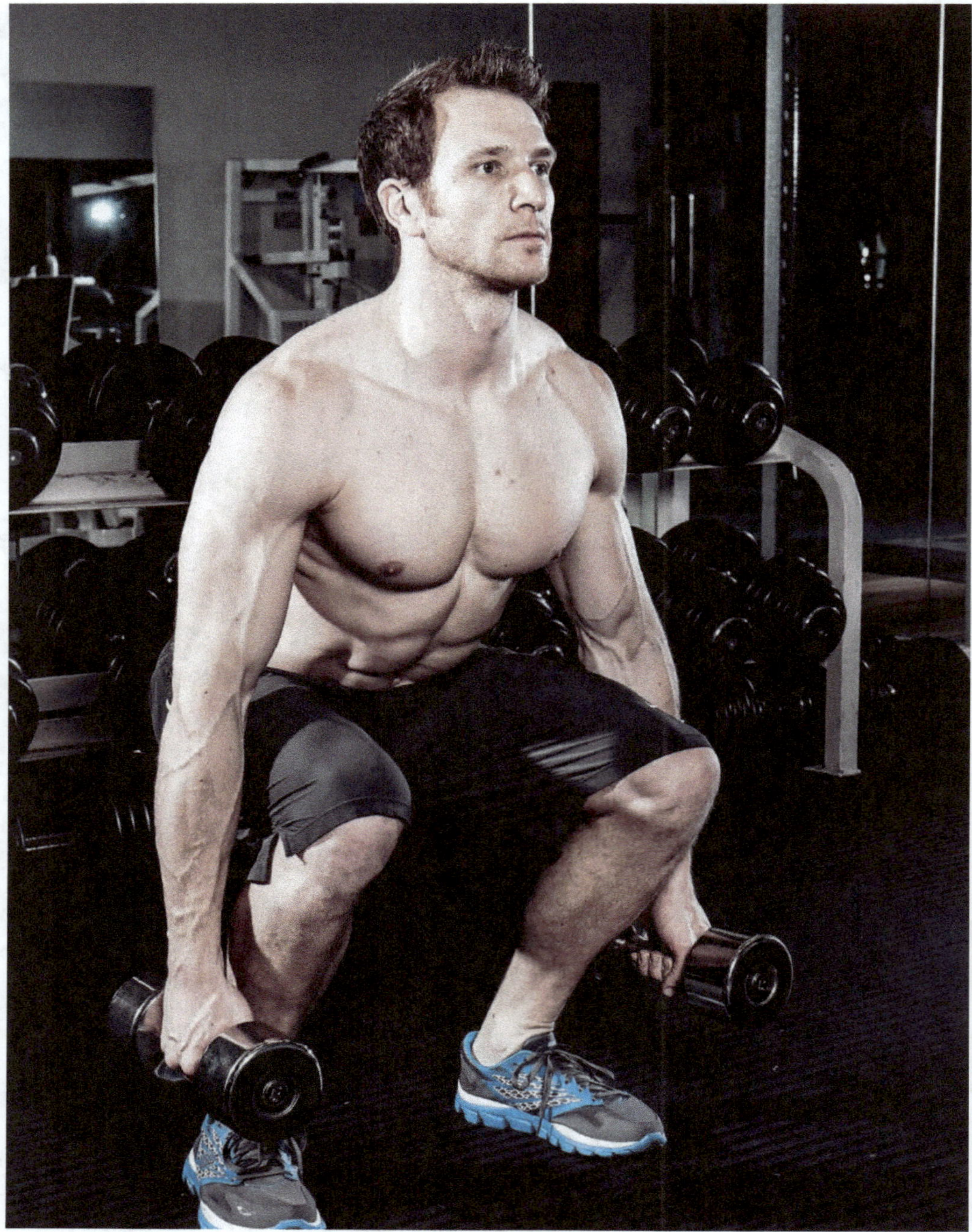

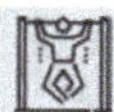

WEEK 1 WORKOUT 1

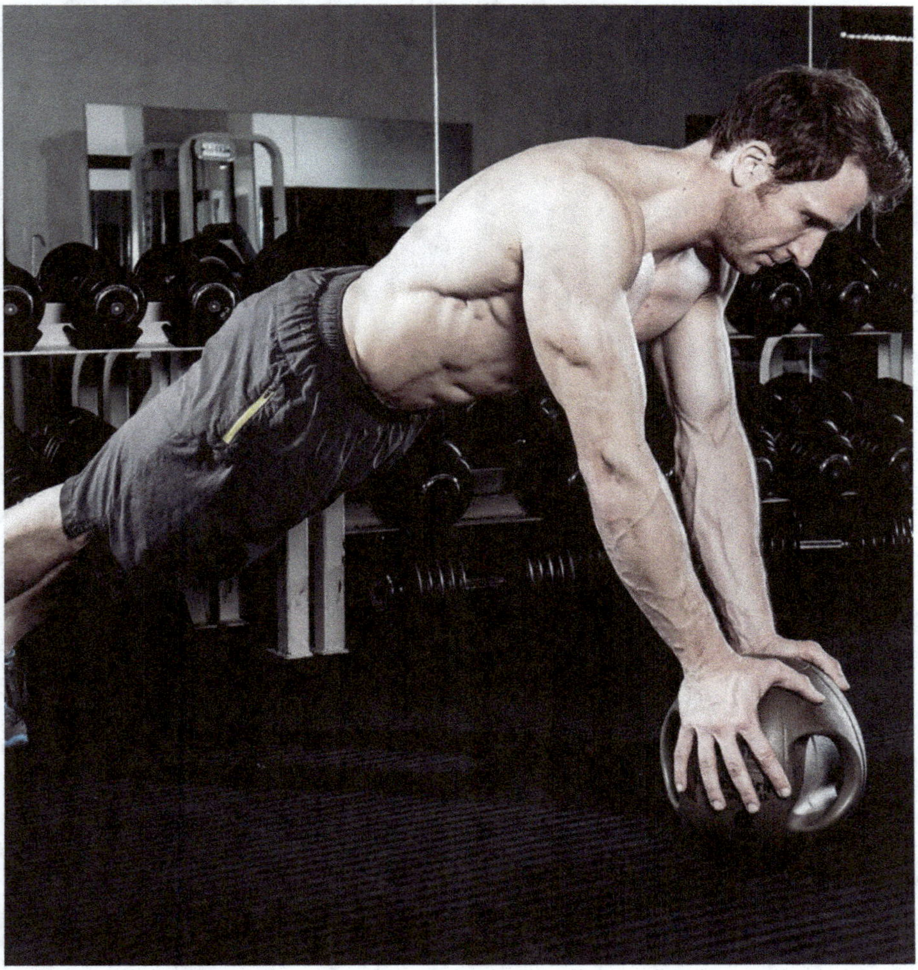

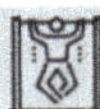

① DUMBBELL BENCH PRESS

SETS 3 **REPS** 12 **TEMPO** 1010 **REST** 60sec

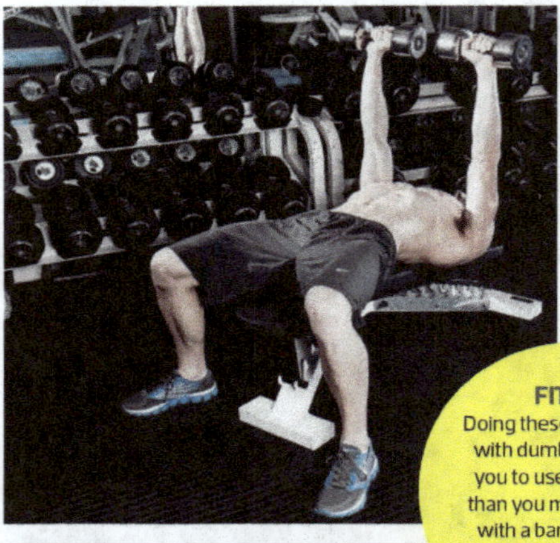

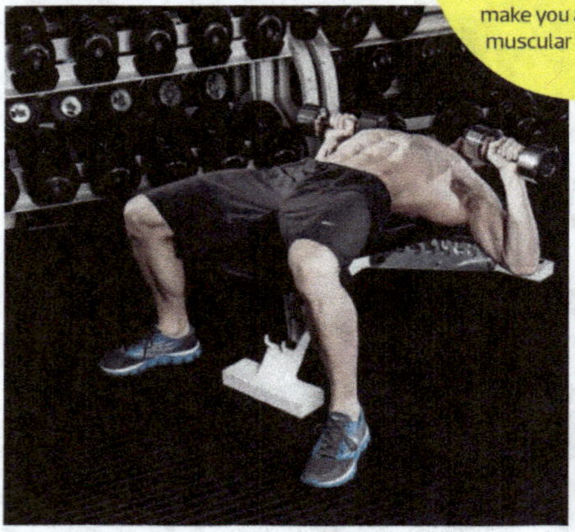

② DB BENT-OVER ROW

SETS 3 **REPS** 12 **TEMPO** 1110 **REST** 60sec

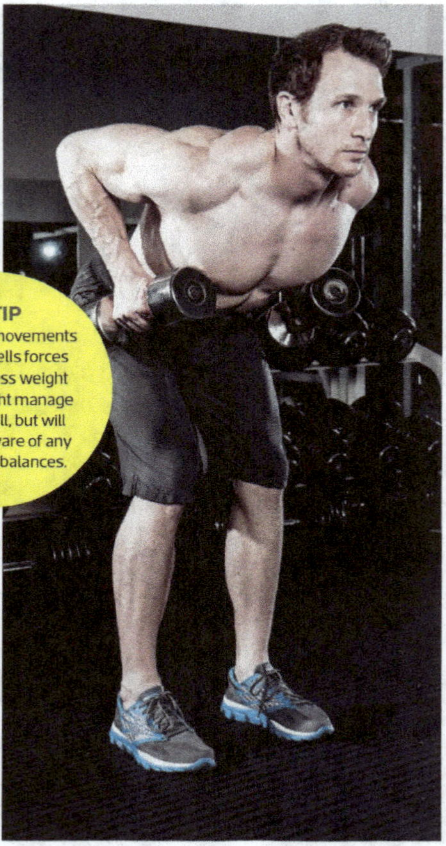

FIT TIP
Doing these movements with dumbbells forces you to use less weight than you might manage with a barbell, but will make you aware of any muscular imbalances.

Lie on a flat bench holding a pair of dumbbells overhead with arms straight. Lower them until you feel a slight stretch in your pecs, then press them overhead, bringing them together until they almost touch.

Holding a pair of dumbbells, bend your knees slightly and lean forwards from the hips. Pull the dumbbells up to your ribcage, retracting your shoulder blades and pulling your elbows behind you. Lower slowly back to the start.

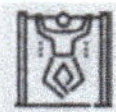

WORKOUT 1

③ DB OVERHEAD PRESS

SETS 3 REPS 12 TEMPO 1010 REST 60sec

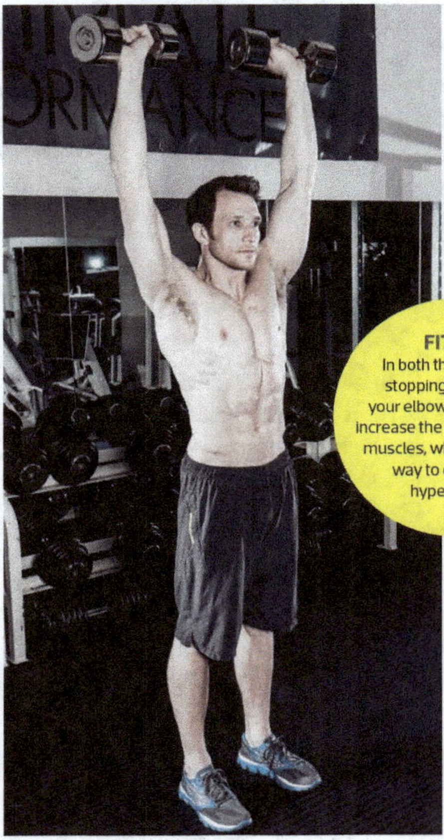

With your feet shoulder-width apart, hold a dumbbell in each hand at shoulder height. Keep your chest up and your core muscles braced. Press the weights directly upwards, until your arms are extended overhead. Then lower slowly.

④ DB BICEPS CURL

SETS 3 REPS 12 TEMPO 1110 REST 60sec

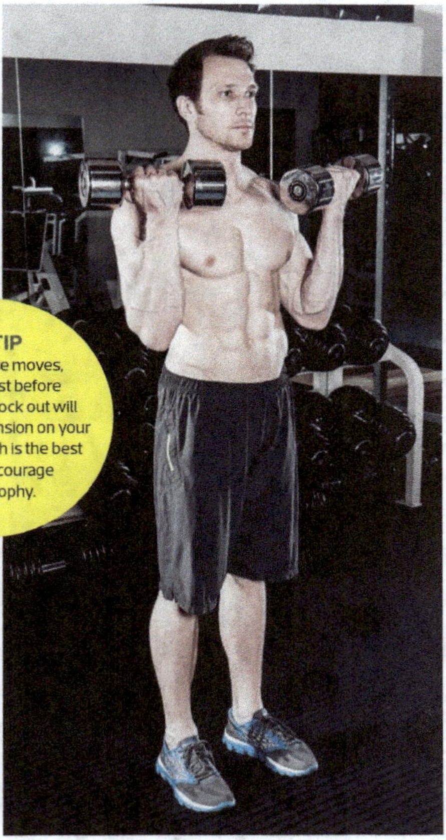

FIT TIP
In both these moves, stopping just before your elbows lock out will increase the tension on your muscles, which is the best way to encourage hypertrophy.

Stand tall holding dumbbells, palms facing away. With your elbows close to your sides, curl the bells towards your chest, stopping just before your forearms are vertical. Squeeze your triceps at the bottom of the move and biceps at the top.

⑤ MED BALL PRESS-UP

SETS 3 REPS 12 TEMPO 1010 REST 60sec

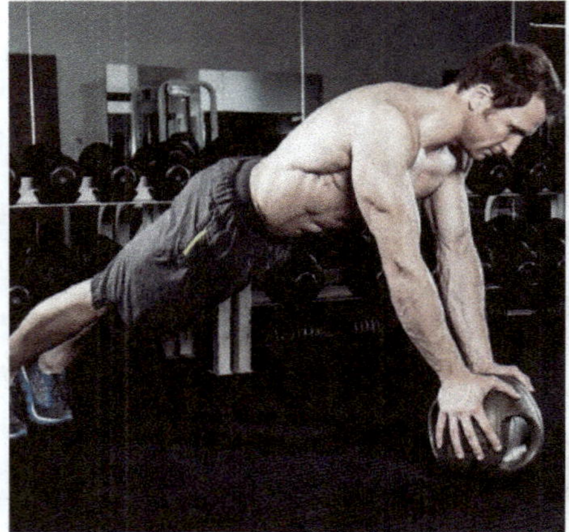

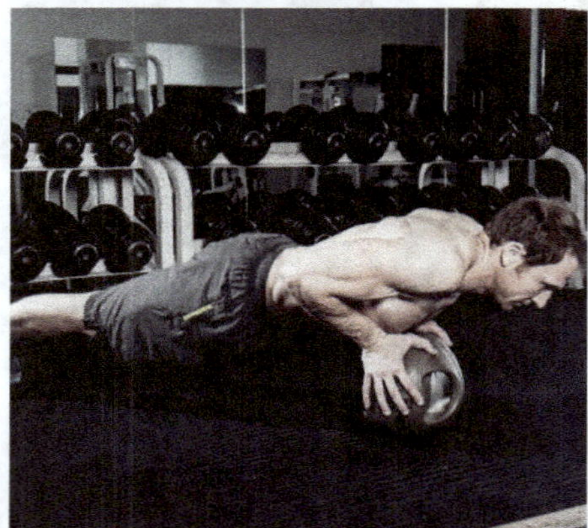

Get into press-up position with your hands on a medicine ball, feet slightly apart. Lower until your chest touches your hands, keeping your elbows as close to your body as possible, then press back up.

⑥ DB ONE-ARM BENT FLYE

SETS 3 REPS 12 each side TEMPO 1110 REST 60sec

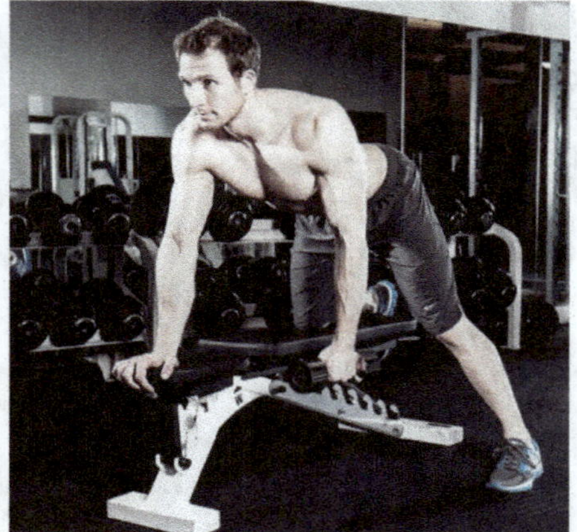

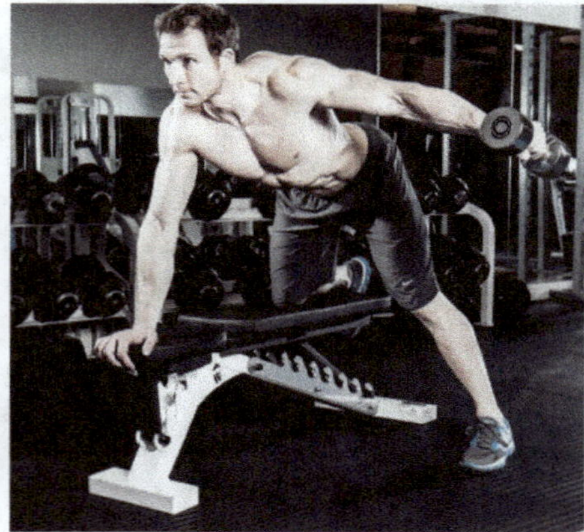

Place one knee on a bench, supporting your torso with a straight arm, holding a dumbbell in the other hand. With your foot flat and core braced, raise the weight to shoulder height, then lower slowly. Do all the reps on one side, then switch.

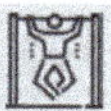

WORKOUT 2

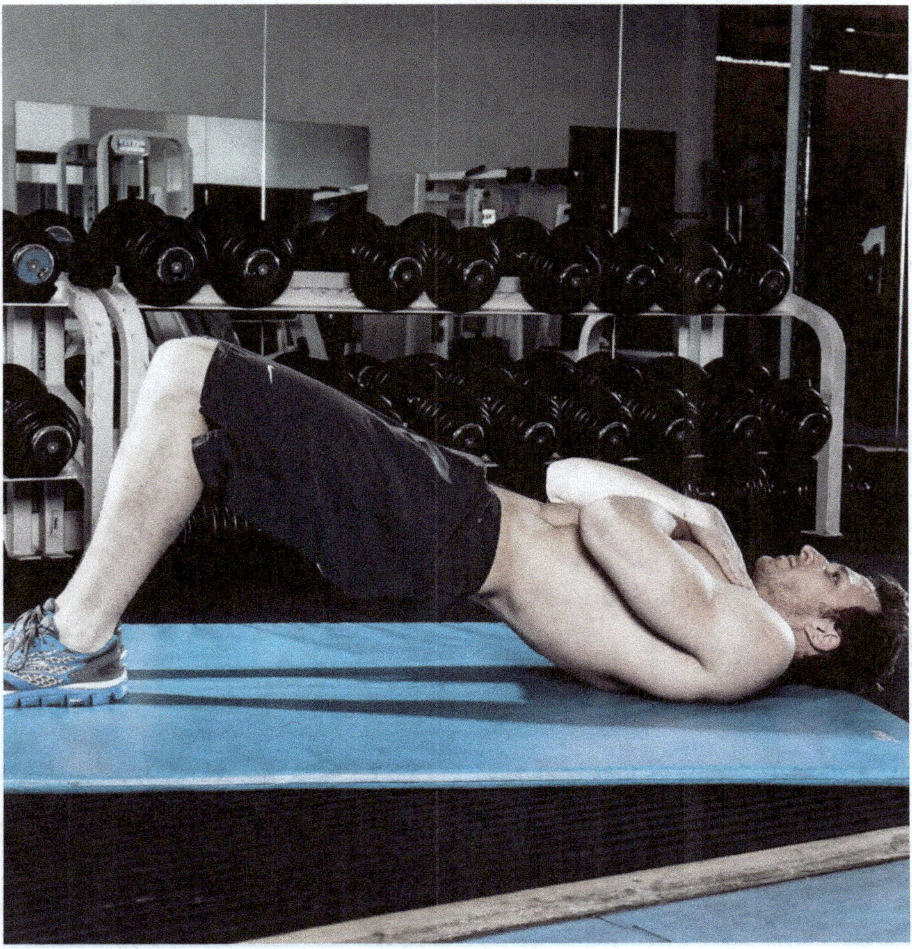

① DB SQUAT

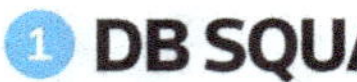

SETS 3 **REPS** 12 **TEMPO** 1010 **REST** 60sec

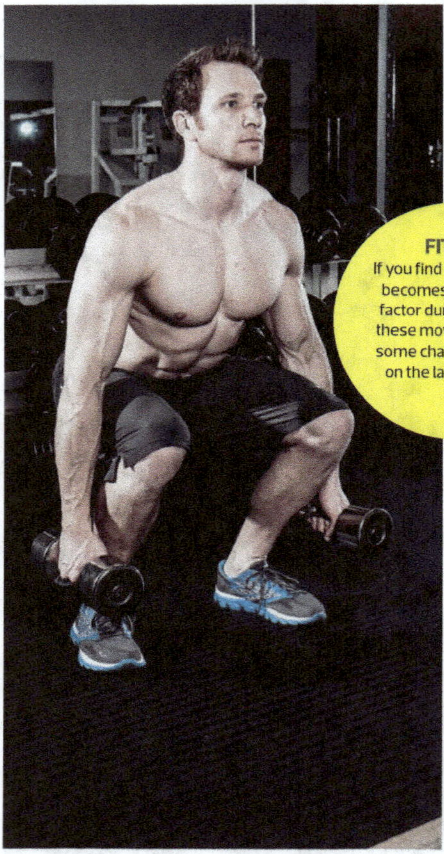

② DB LUNGE

SETS 3 **REPS** 12 each side **TEMPO** 1010 **REST** 60sec

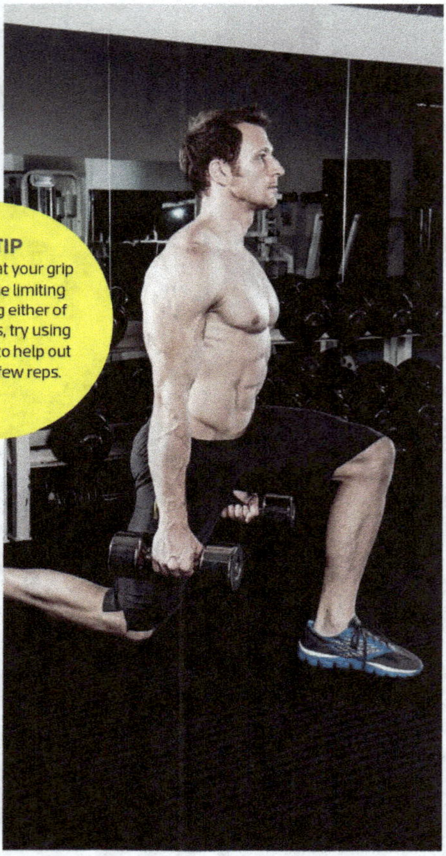

FIT TIP
If you find that your grip becomes the limiting factor during either of these moves, try using some chalk to help out on the last few reps.

Holding a pair of dumbbells, sit down and back into a squat. Your thighs should be parallel to the floor at the bottom of the move. Keep your weight on your heels as you drive back up.

Holding a dumbbell in each hand, take one step forwards and lower your body until both knees are bent at right angles. Then push off your front foot to reverse the movement.

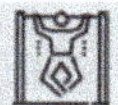

WORKOUT 2

③ DB ROMANIAN DEADLIFT

SETS 3 **REPS** 12 **TEMPO** 1110 **REST** 60sec

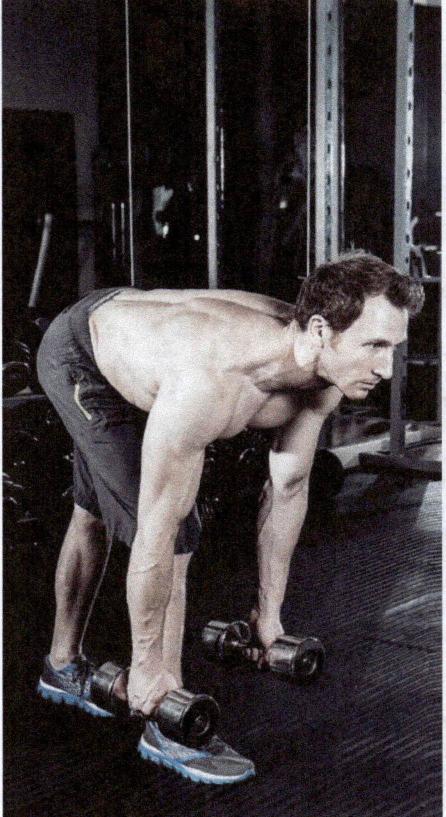

Holding a set of dumbbells and keeping a slight bend in your knees, bend forwards from the hips and lower the dumbbells until you feel a stretch in your hamstrings. Reverse the move back to the start and push your hips forwards.

④ GLUTE BRIDGE

SETS 3 **REPS** 12 **TEMPO** 1110 **REST** 60sec

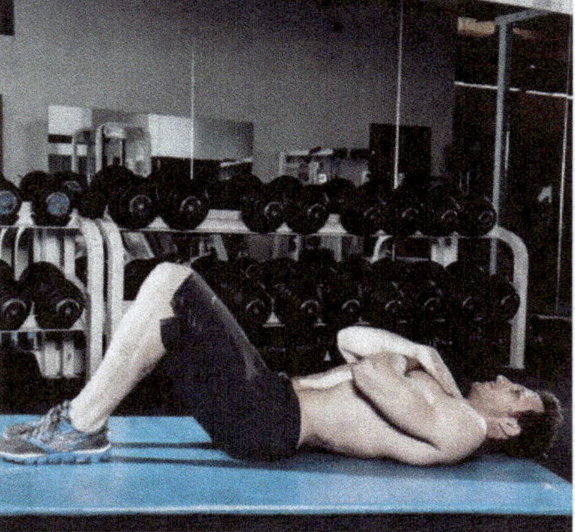

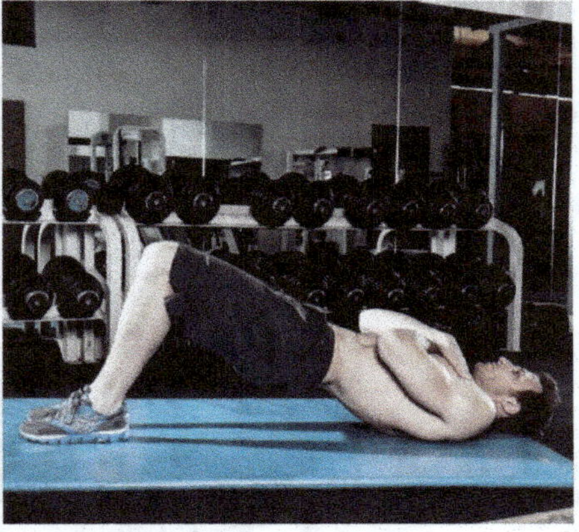

Lie on the floor with your feet close to your glutes. Drive through your heels to raise your hips, tense your glutes at the top of the move, then lower under control. If it's too easy, add a weight plate.

⑤ DB SIDE LUNGE

SETS 3 **REPS** 12 each side **TEMPO** 1010 **REST** 60sec

Holding a pair of dumbbells, take a big step out to one side, leaving your trailing leg straight as you bend your leading leg. Push off your foot to return to the start position and repeat on the other side.

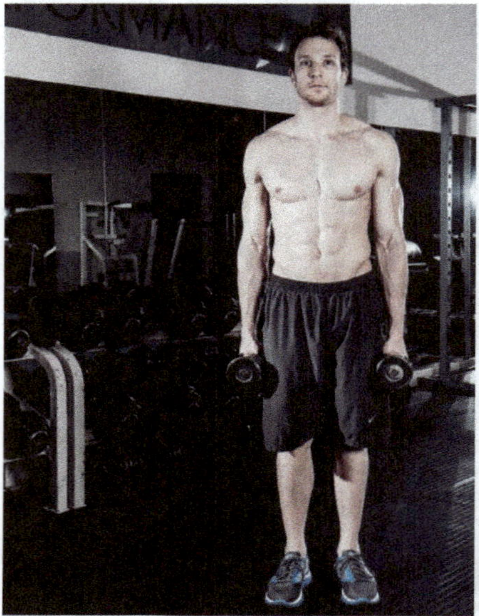

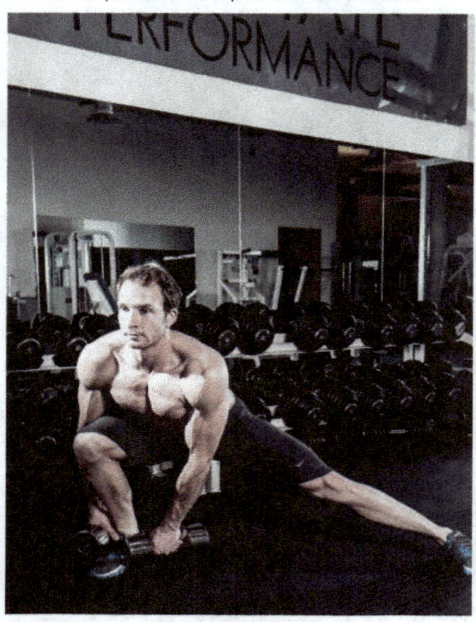

⑥ PLANK

SETS 3 **TIME** 30sec **TEMPO** N/A **REST** 60sec

Get into a plank position with your forearms on the floor and hands clasped in front of you. Brace your abs and glutes to keep your body in a straight line. Hold that position.

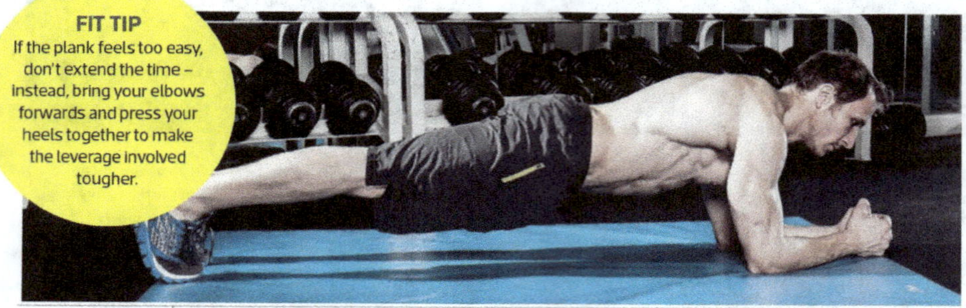

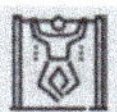

WORKOUT 3

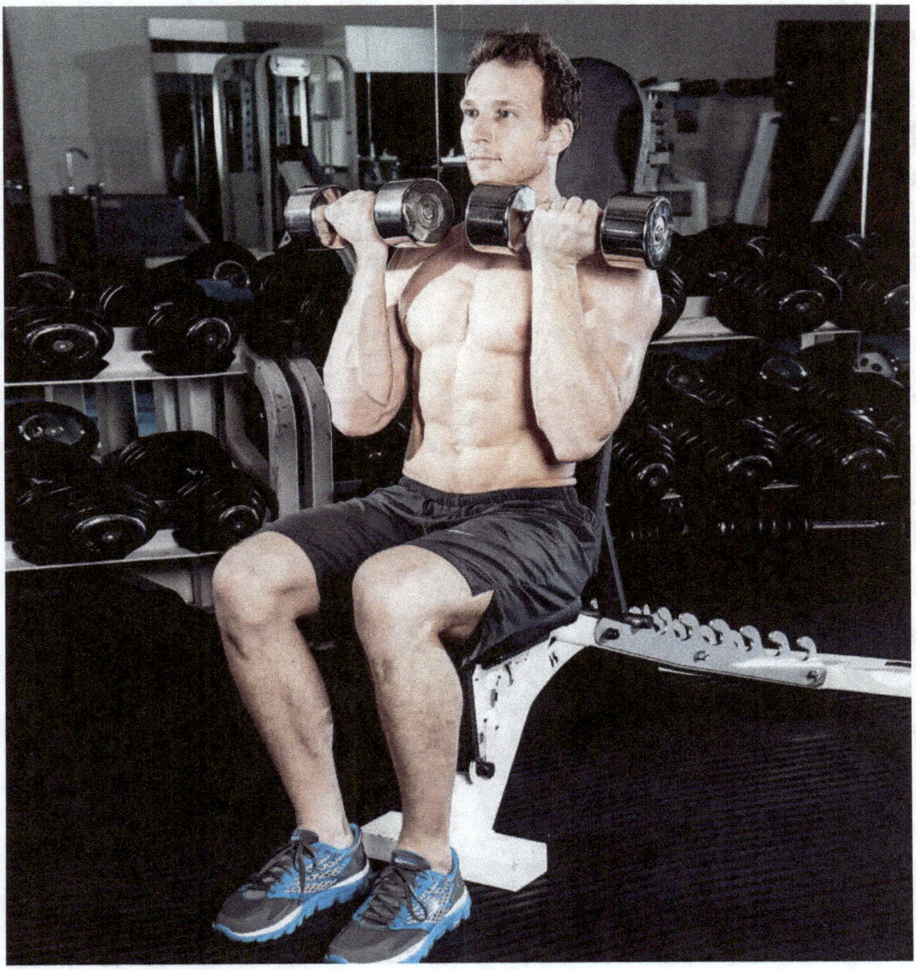

① INCLINE DB BENCH PRESS

SETS 3 REPS 12 TEMPO 1010 REST 60sec

② DB ONE-ARM ROW

SETS 3 REPS 12 each side TEMPO 1110 REST 60sec

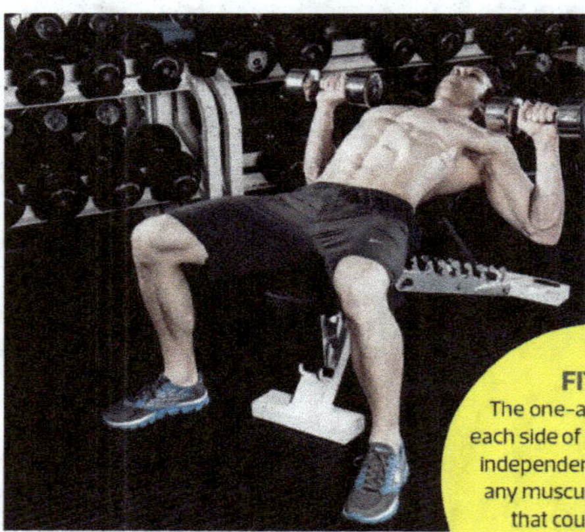

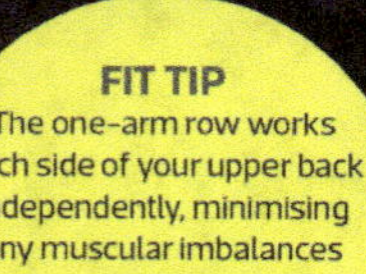

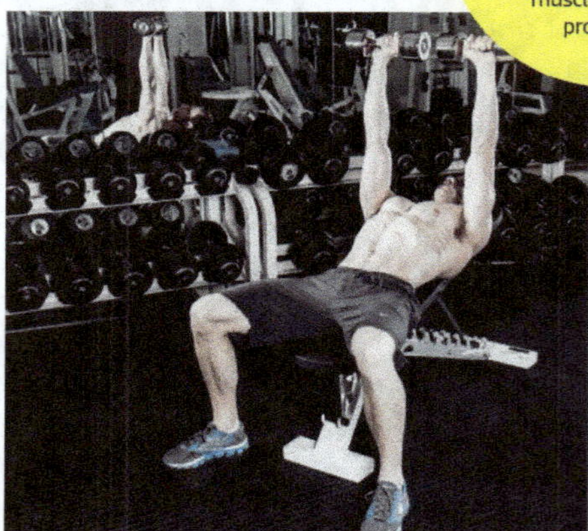

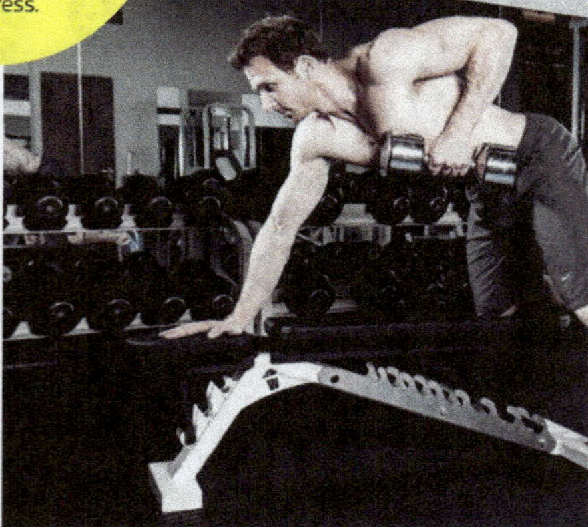

Lie on a bench set at a 30° angle holding a dumbbell in each hand. Keep your feet flat on the floor and your back against the bench. Press the weights straight up, without locking out at the top, then lower.

Place one knee on a bench, supporting your torso with a straight arm, holding a dumbbell in the other hand. With your foot flat and core braced, row the weight up, leading with your elbow, then lower. Do all the reps on one side, then switch.

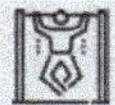

WORKOUT 3

③ DB ARNOLD PRESS

SETS 3 REPS 12 TEMPO 1010 REST 60sec

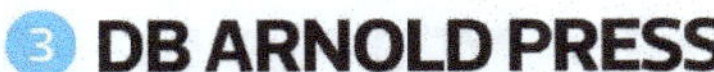

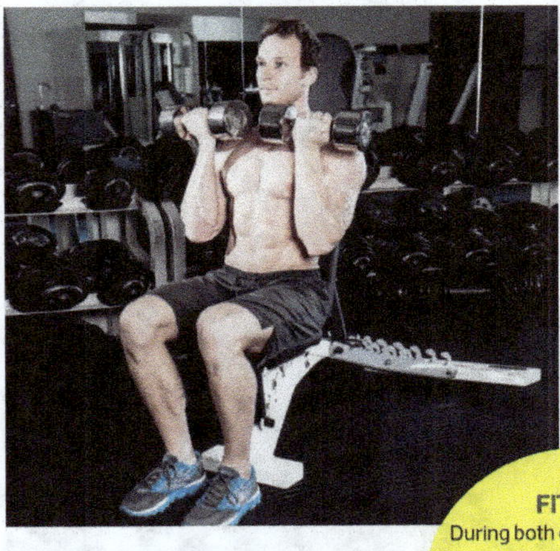

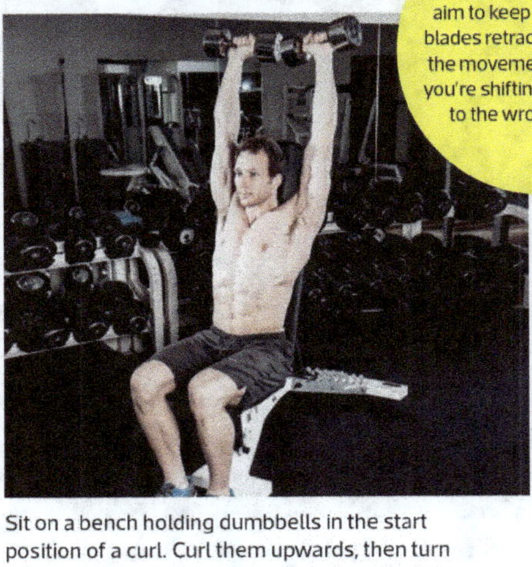

Sit on a bench holding dumbbells in the start position of a curl. Curl them upwards, then turn your palms away and press them overhead. Then reverse the whole movement to complete the rep.

④ DB LATERAL RAISE

SETS 3 REPS 12 TEMPO 1110 REST 60sec

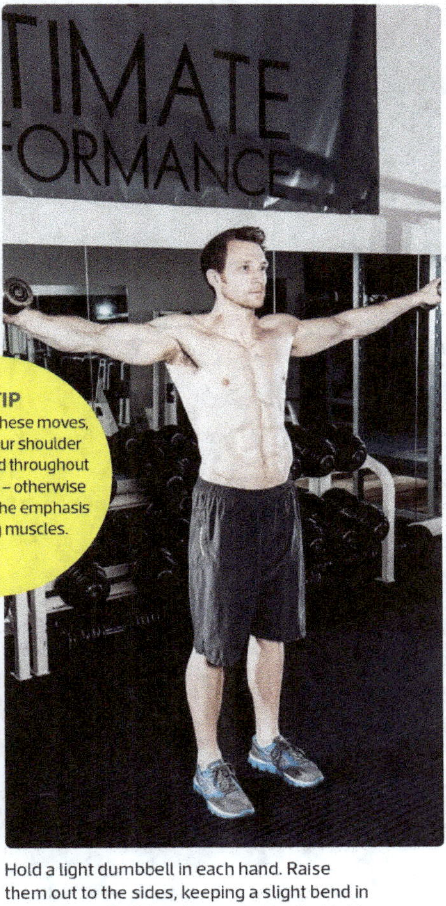

FIT TIP
During both of these moves, aim to keep your shoulder blades retracted throughout the movement – otherwise you're shifting the emphasis to the wrong muscles.

Hold a light dumbbell in each hand. Raise them out to the sides, keeping a slight bend in your elbows. To keep the tension on the right muscles, keep your pinkies higher than your thumbs and don't go above shoulder height.

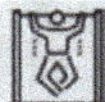

⑤ DB HAMMER CURL

SETS 3 REPS 12 TEMPO 1110 REST 60sec

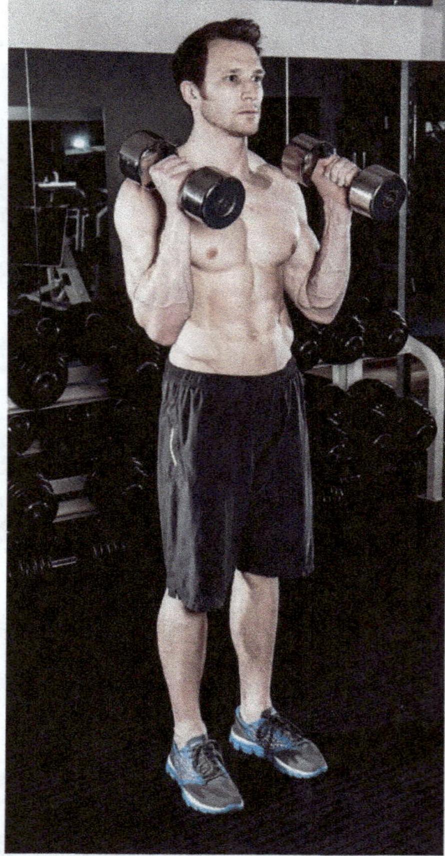

Start by holding dumbbells, palms facing your thighs. Curl both weights up, squeezing your biceps at the top of the move. Don't alternate arms - this takes too much tension off the muscle while one arm rests.

⑥ DIAMOND PRESS-UP

SETS 3 REPS 12 TEMPO 1010 REST 60sec

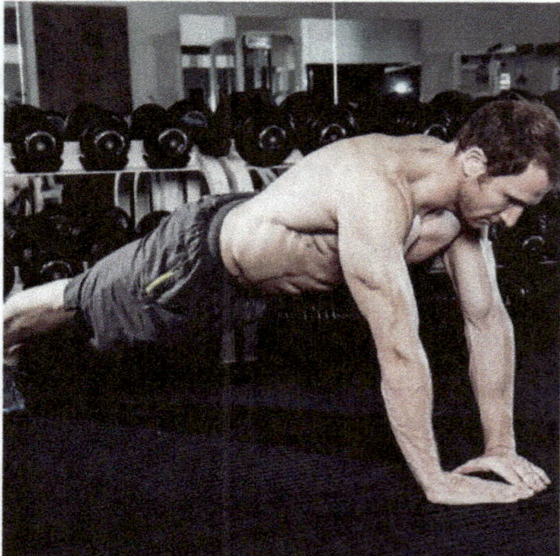

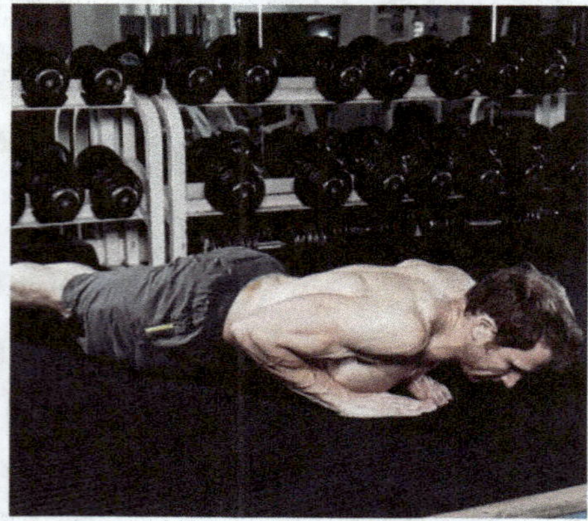

Get in a press-up position but with your hands in a diamond – the tips of your thumbs and index fingers together – and lower your chest until it touches your hands. Keep your elbows tucked as you press back up.

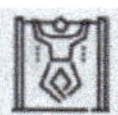

WORKOUT 4

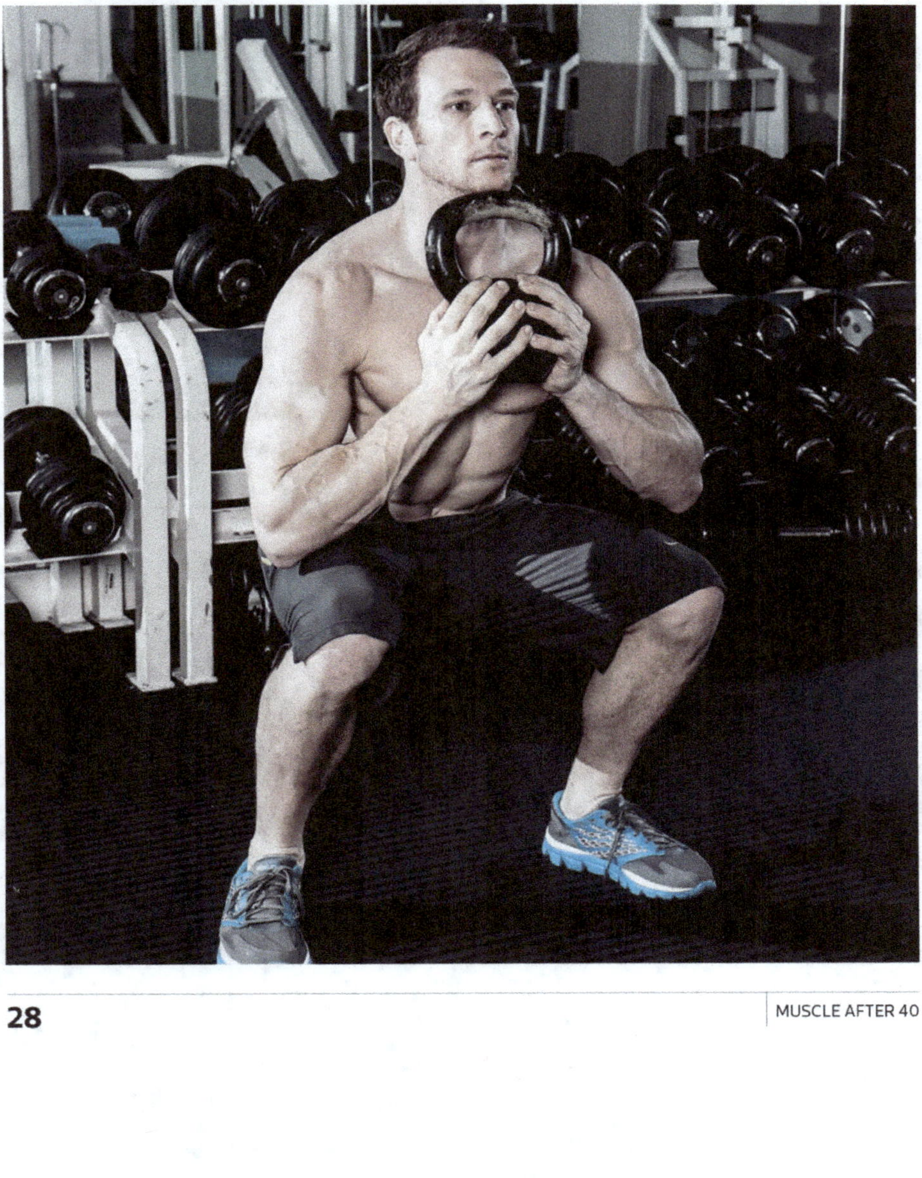

① LYING LEG CURL

SETS 3 REPS 12 TEMPO 1010 REST 60sec

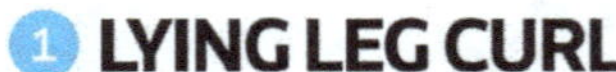

② LEG PRESS

SETS 3 REPS 12 TEMPO 1010 REST 60sec

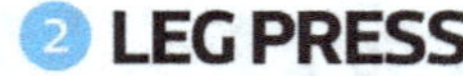

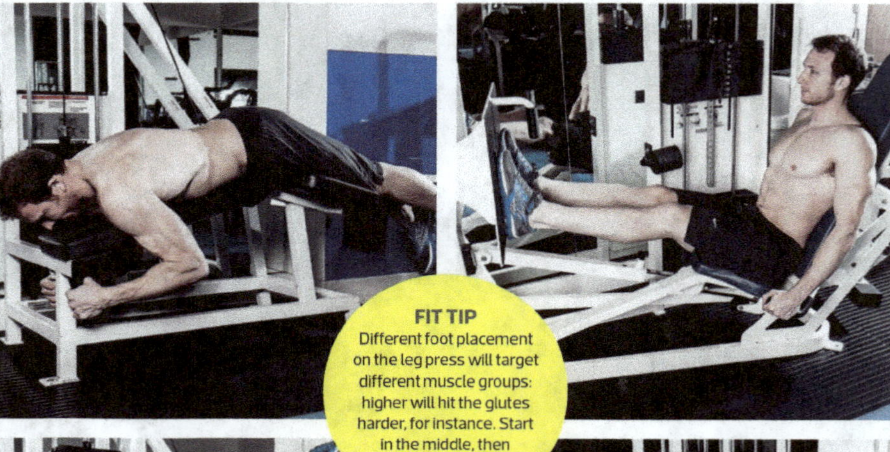

FIT TIP
Different foot placement on the leg press will target different muscle groups: higher will hit the glutes harder, for instance. Start in the middle, then experiment.

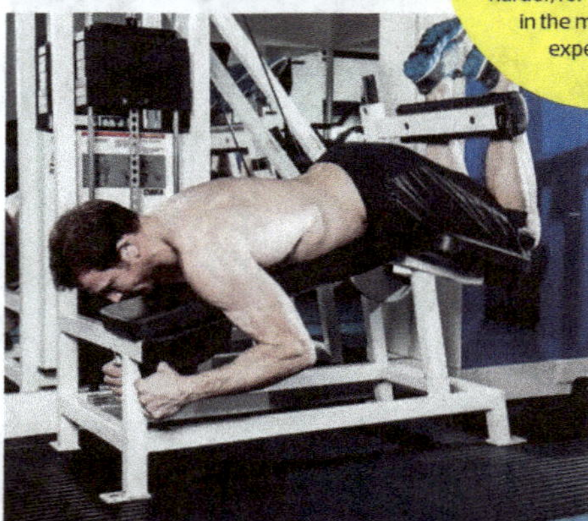

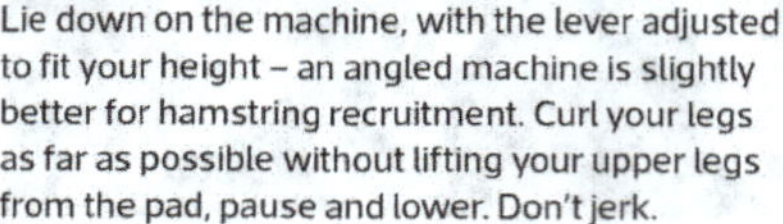

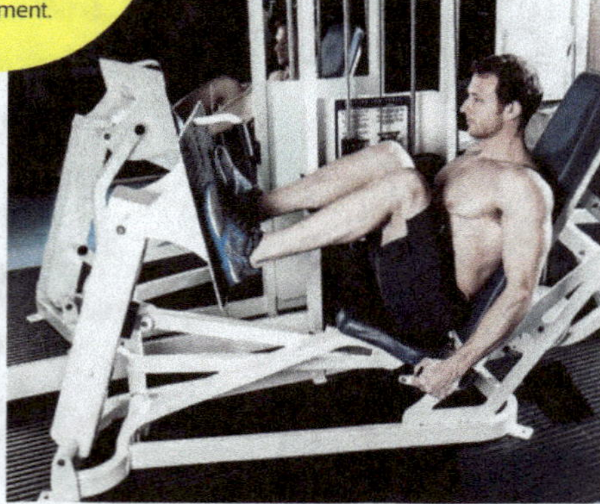

Lie down on the machine, with the lever adjusted to fit your height – an angled machine is slightly better for hamstring recruitment. Curl your legs as far as possible without lifting your upper legs from the pad, pause and lower. Don't jerk.

Sit on the machine, release the lock, and then slowly lower the platform until your legs are at 90°. Pause briefly at the bottom, then push through your heels to straighten your legs. Don't lock out fully at the top.

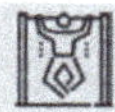

WORKOUT 4

③ SEATED CALF RAISE

SETS 3 **REPS** 12 **TEMPO** 1010 **REST** 60sec

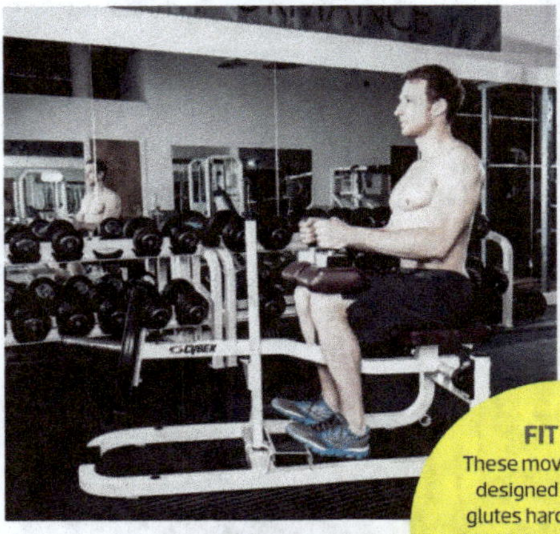

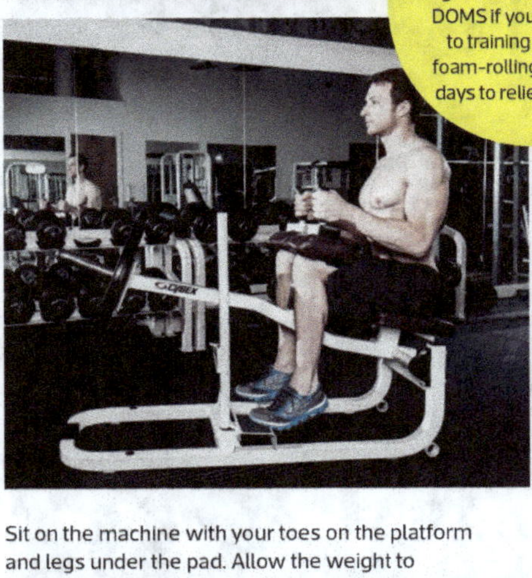

④ DB REVERSE LUNGE

SETS 3 **REPS** 12 each side **TEMPO** 1010 **REST** 60sec

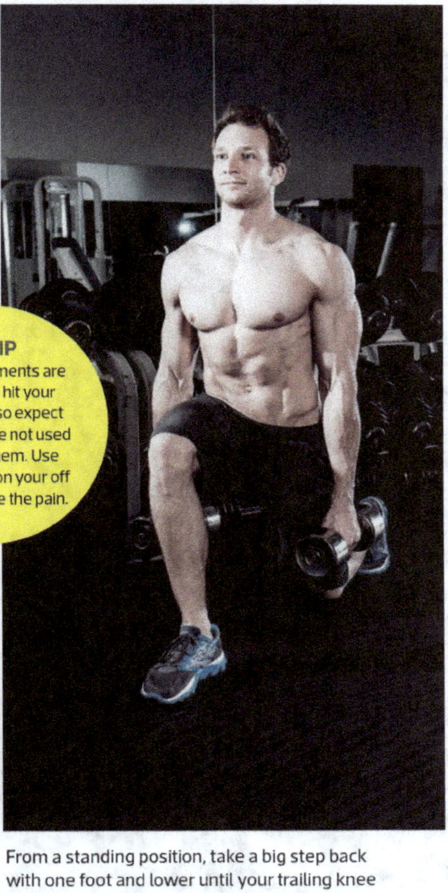

FIT TIP
These movements are designed to hit your glutes hard, so expect DOMS if you're not used to training them. Use foam-rolling on your off days to relieve the pain.

Sit on the machine with your toes on the platform and legs under the pad. Allow the weight to descend until you feel a stretch in your calves, pause, then raise your heels by bringing your ankles as high as possible. Pause and repeat.

From a standing position, take a big step back with one foot and lower until your trailing knee brushes the floor. Stand up, and repeat on the other side. This lunge variation makes it easier to maintain good knee alignment.

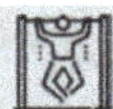

5 GOBLET SQUAT

SETS 3 **REPS** 12 **TEMPO** 1010 **REST** 60sec

Stand with your feet shoulder-width apart holding a dumbbell or kettlebell like a drinking goblet. Keeping your core braced, squat until you can touch your knees with your elbows. Drive up through your heels to return to the start position.

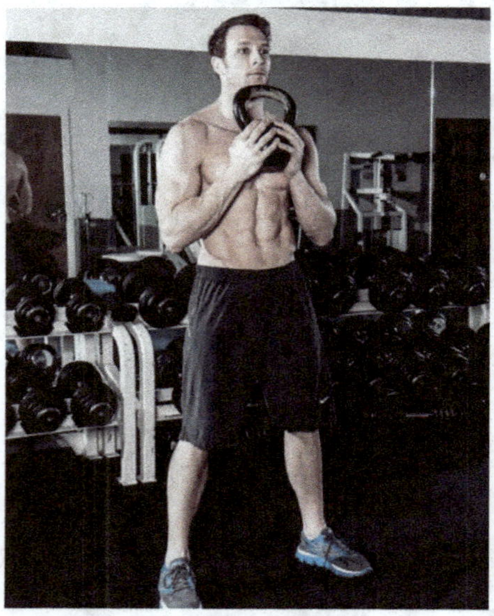

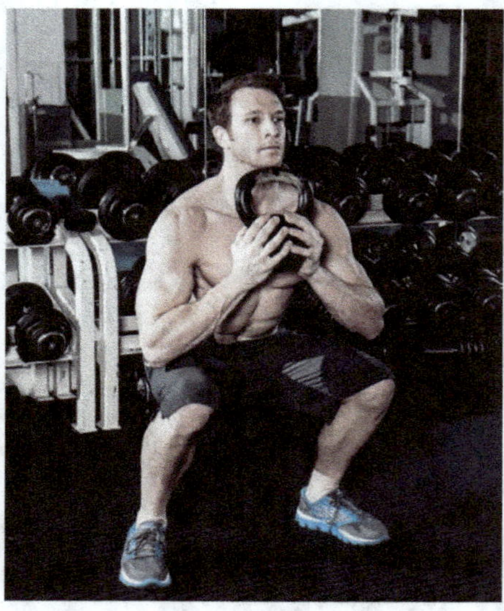

6 PLANK

SETS 3 **TIME** 45sec **REST** 60sec

Get into a plank position with your forearms on the floor and hands clasped in front of you, then brace your abs and glutes to keep your body in a straight line. Hold that position.

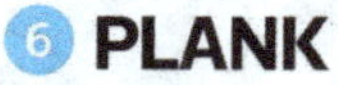

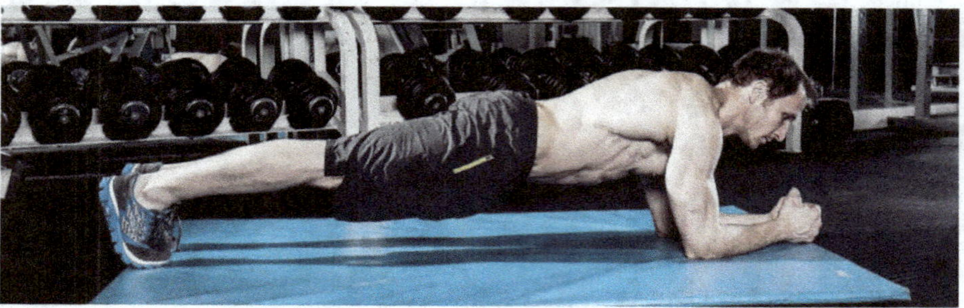

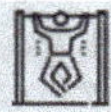

WEEK 2

Drop the reps but up your sets, and you'll increase your work capacity

WORKOUT 1 **UPPER BODY 1**

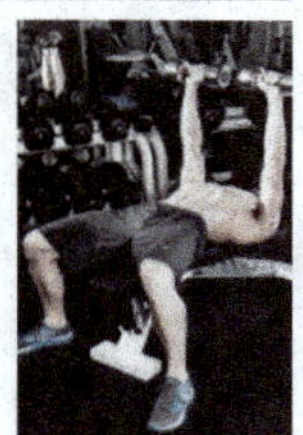

EXERCISE	SETS	REPS	TEMPO	REST
1 Dumbbell bench press	4	10	1010	60SEC
2 Dumbbell bent-over row	4	10	1110	60SEC
3 Dumbbell overhead press	4	10	1010	60SEC
4 Dumbbell biceps curl	4	10	1110	60SEC
5 Medicine ball press-up	4	10	1010	60SEC
6 Dumbbell one-arm bent-over flye	4	10	1110	60SEC

WORKOUT 2 **LOWER BODY 1**

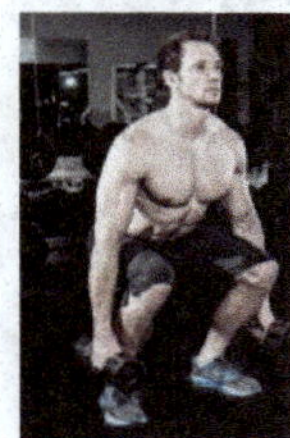

EXERCISE	SETS	REPS/TIME	TEMPO	REST
1 Dumbbell squat	4	10	1010	60SEC
2 Dumbbell lunge	4	10 EACH SIDE	1010	60SEC
3 Dumbbell Romanian deadlift	4	10	1110	60SEC
4 Glute bridge	4	10	1110	60SEC
5 Dumbbell side lunge	4	10 EACH SIDE	1010	60SEC
6 Plank	4	30SEC	N/A	60SEC

WORKOUT 3 **UPPER BODY 2**

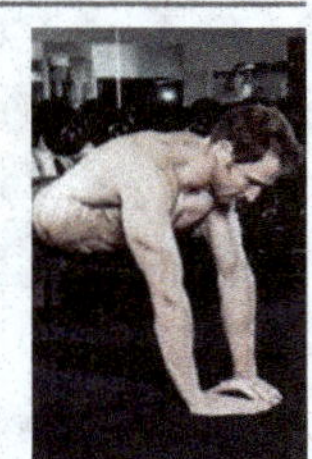

EXERCISE	SETS	REPS	TEMPO	REST
1 Incline dumbbell bench press	4	10	1010	60SEC
2 Dumbbell one-arm bent-over row	4	10	1110	60SEC
3 Dumbbell Arnold press	4	10	1010	60SEC
4 Dumbbell lateral raise	4	10	1110	60SEC
5 Dumbbell hammer curl	4	10	1110	60SEC
6 Diamond press-up	4	10	1010	60SEC

WORKOUT 4 **LOWER BODY 2**

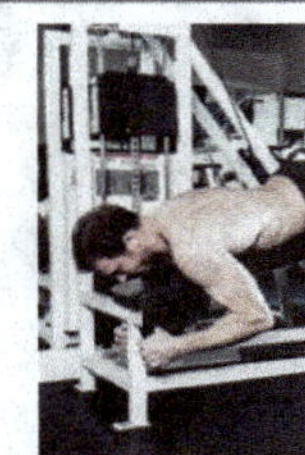

EXERCISE	SETS	REPS/TIME	TEMPO	REST
1 Leg curl	4	10	1010	60SEC
2 Leg press	4	10	1010	60SEC
3 Seated calf raise	4	10	1010	60SEC
4 Dumbbell reverse lunge	4	10 EACH SIDE	1010	60SEC
5 Goblet squat	4	10	1010	60SEC
6 Plank	4	30SEC	N/A	60SEC

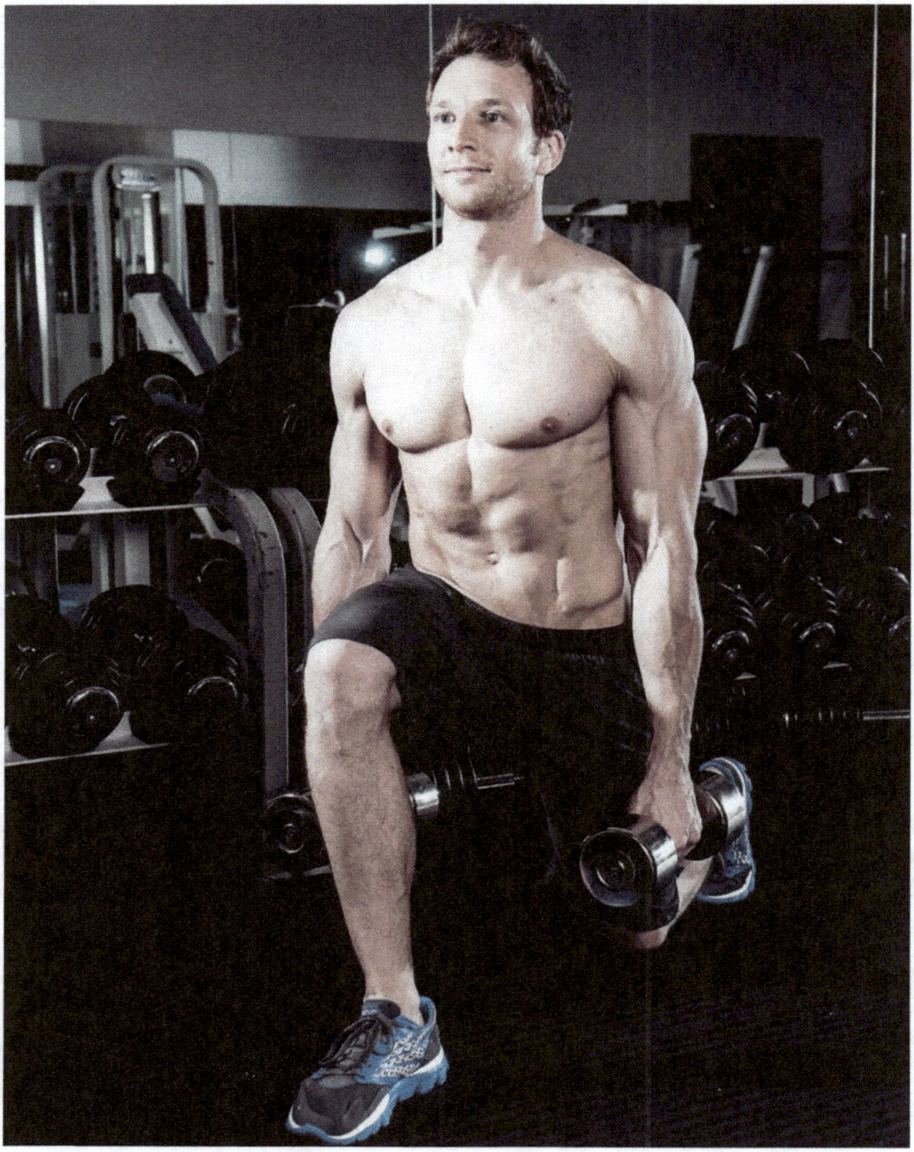

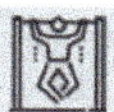

WEEK 3 WORKOUT 1

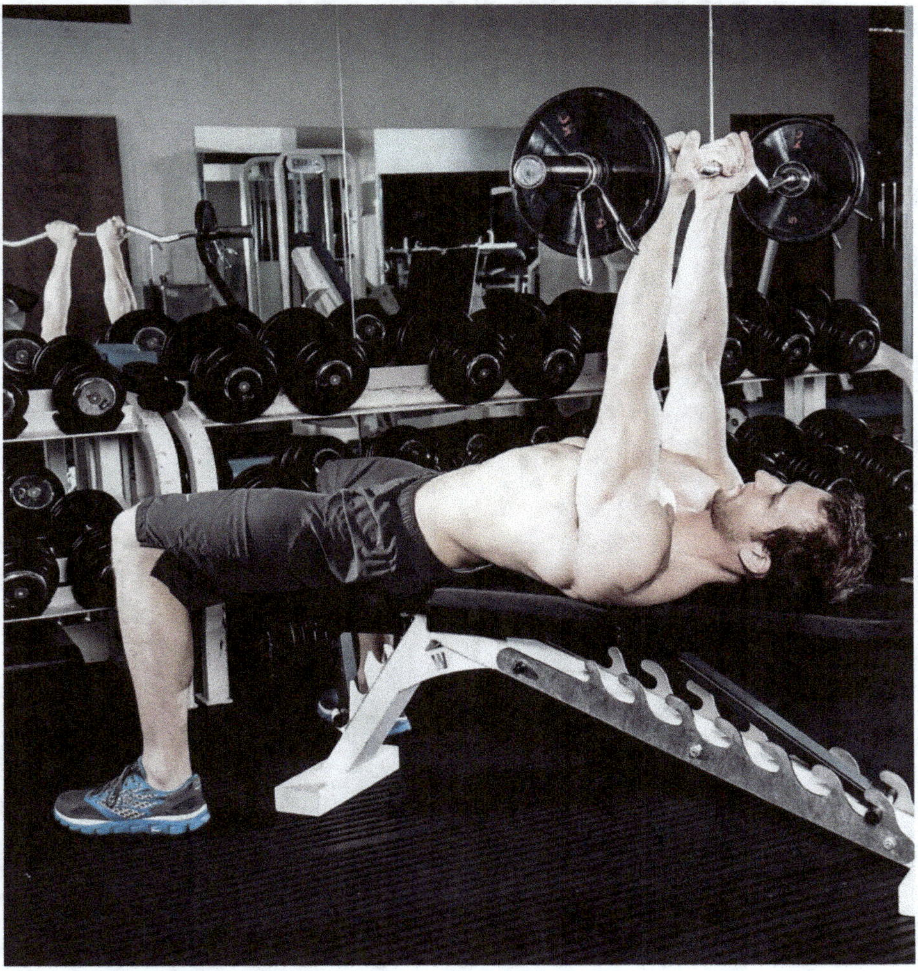

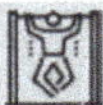

① BENCH PRESS

SETS 3 REPS 12 TEMPO 1010 REST 60sec

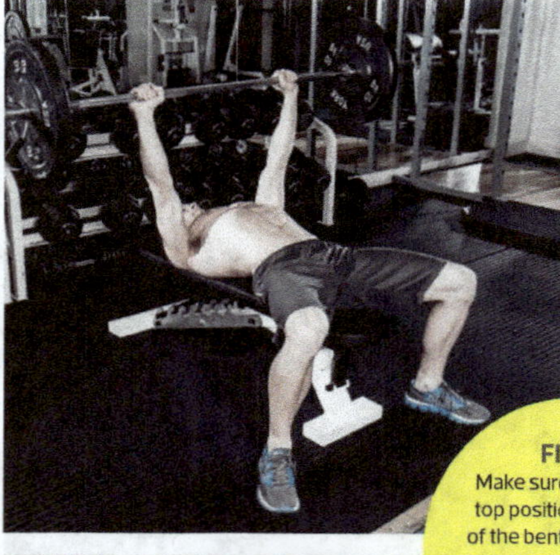

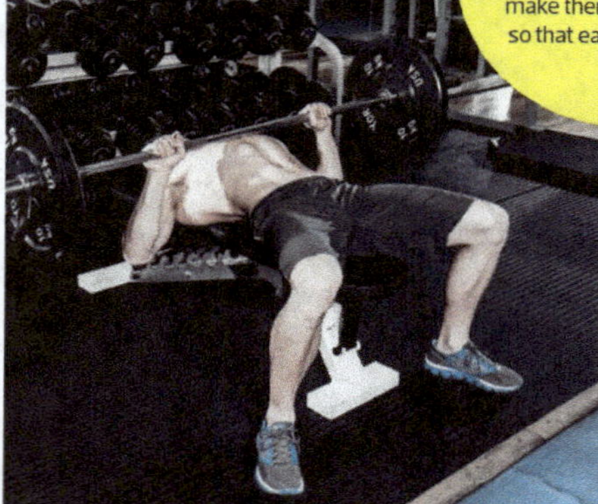

Lie on the bench with your feet on the floor. Hold the bar with your hands shoulder-width apart. Slowly lower the bar to your chest. Drive your feet hard into the floor and push the bar back strongly to the start position.

② BENT-OVER ROW

SETS 3 REPS 12 TEMPO 1110 REST 60sec

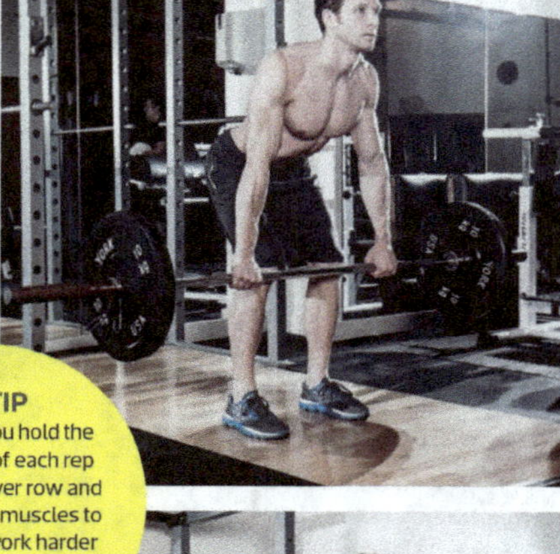

FIT TIP
Make sure you hold the top position of each rep of the bent-over row and squeeze your muscles to make them work harder so that each rep counts.

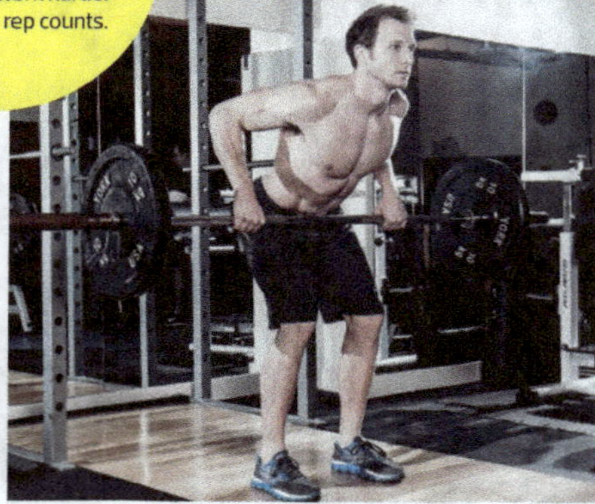

Bend your knees slightly and lean forwards with your hands just wider than shoulder-width apart on the bar. Pull the bar up to your lower sternum, focusing on pulling your elbows behind you, then lower under control.

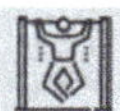

WORKOUT 1

③ OVERHEAD PRESS

SETS 3 REPS 12 TEMPO 1010 REST 60sec

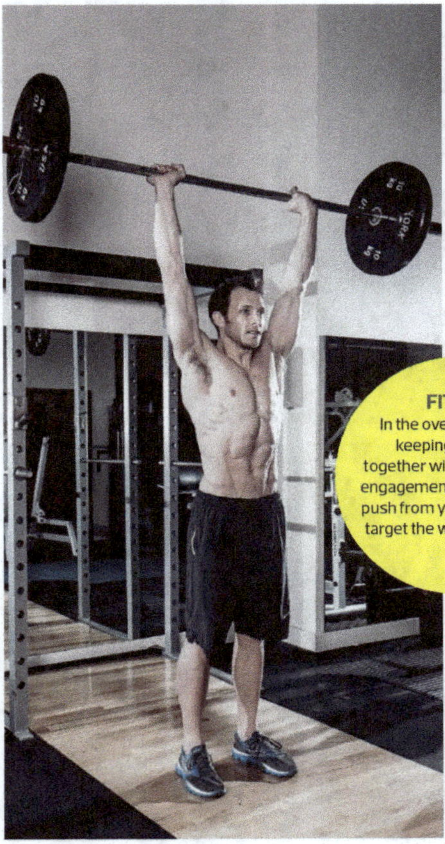

FIT TIP
In the overhead press, keeping your feet together will increase core engagement. Don't use any push from your legs – you'll target the wrong muscles.

Hold the bar with your thumbs wrapped on the same side as your fingers, touching your shoulders. Brace your glutes and core and press the bar overhead, putting your head through the 'window' of your arms at the top. Lower under control.

④ LYING DB PULL-OVER

SETS 3 REPS 12 TEMPO 1010 REST 60sec

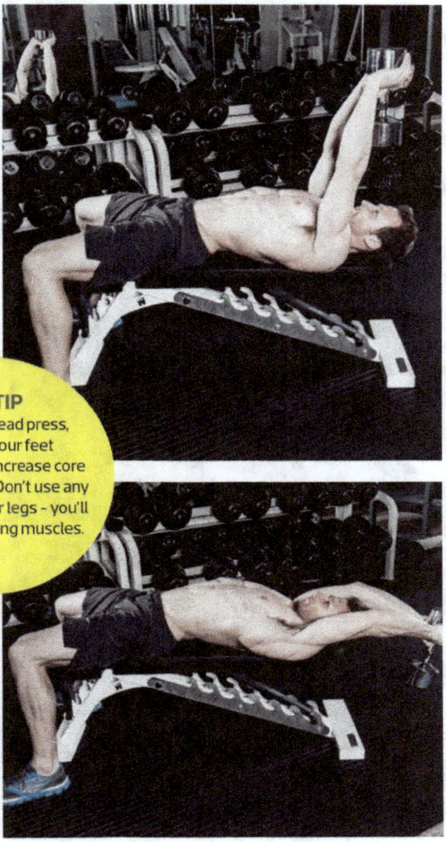

Lie on a bench with a dumbbell in both hands, directly above your head. Let the dumbbell descend behind your head, with your arms fairly straight. Pause, then 'pull' it back up to the start position.

⑤ EZ-BAR BICEPS CURL

SETS 3 REPS 12 TEMPO 1010 REST 60sec

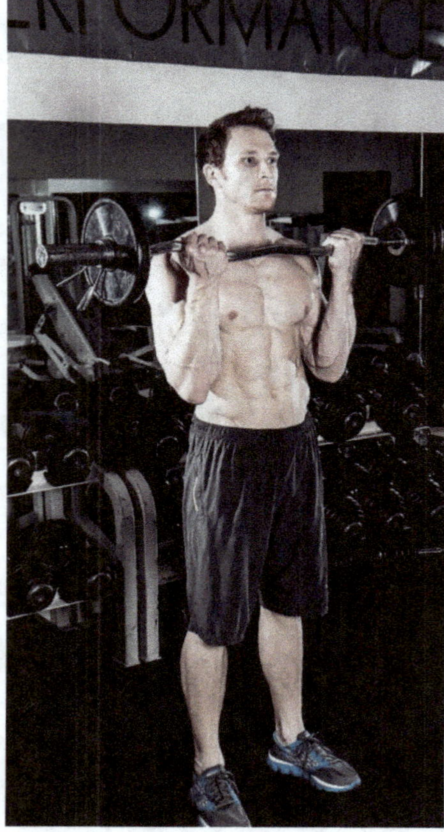

Using an EZ-bar reduces stress on your elbows. Stand straight and curl the bar upwards. Squeeze your biceps at the top of the movement and your triceps at the bottom.

⑥ LYING EZ-BAR EXTENSION

SETS 3 REPS 12 TEMPO 1010 REST 60sec

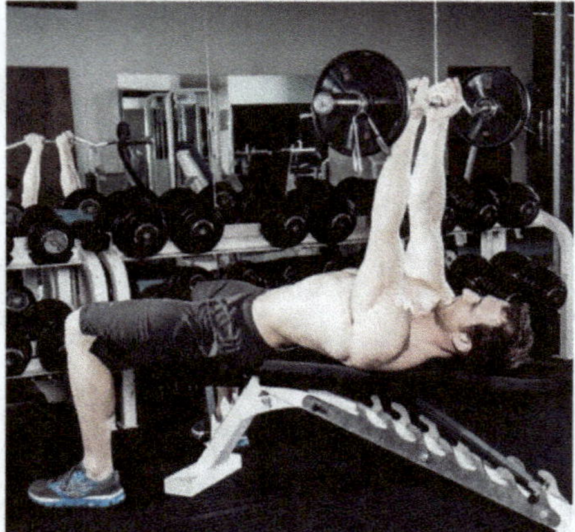

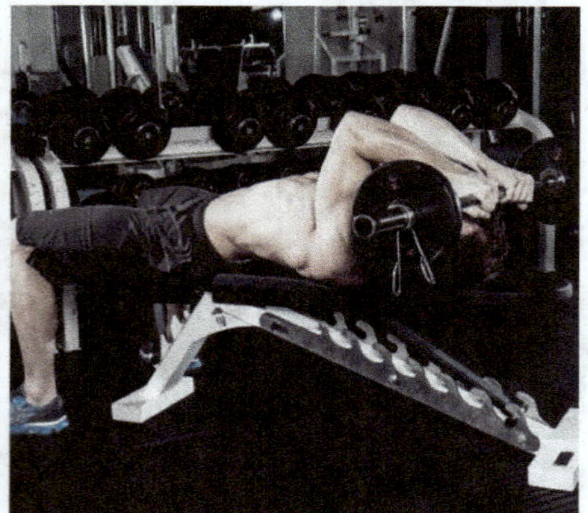

Lie on a bench, holding an EZ-bar above your chest with straight arms. Slowly lower the bar towards the top of your head by bending your elbows, which should stay pointing directly to the ceiling. Then straighten your arms.

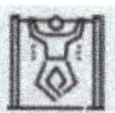

WORKOUT 2

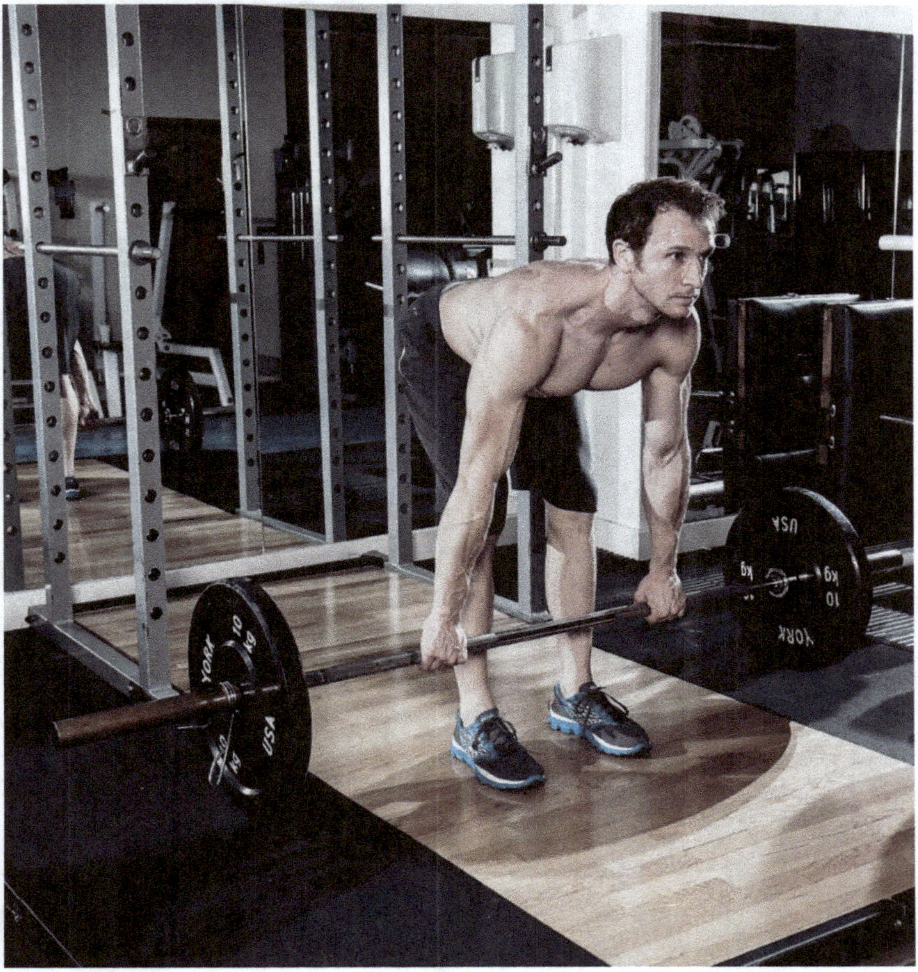

① BARBELL SQUAT

SETS 3 REPS 12 TEMPO 1010 REST 60sec

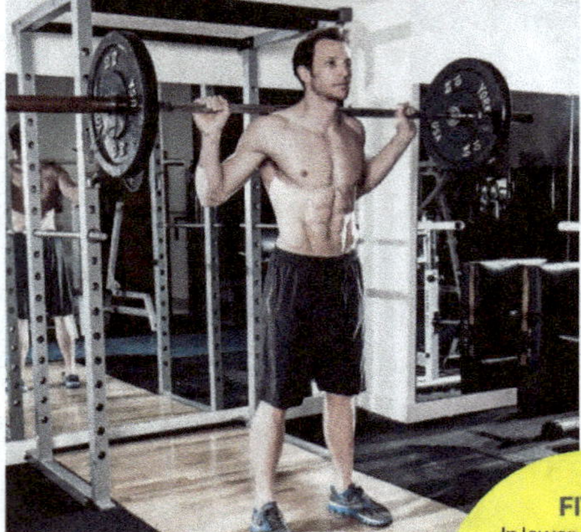

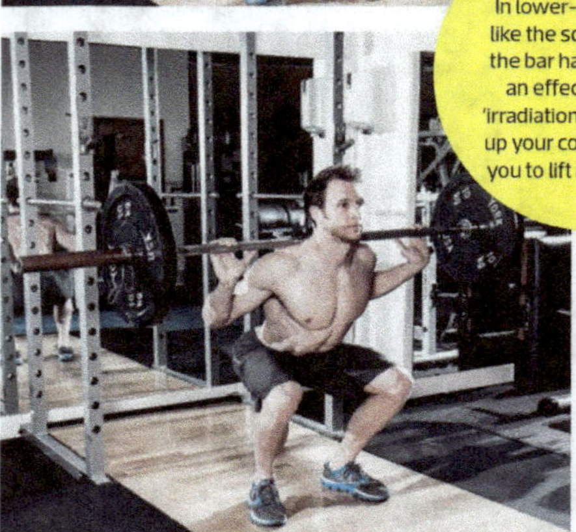

Stand with your feet just wider than shoulder-width apart, holding the bar on your upper traps. Sit down and back, keeping your chest up and your core engaged. When you've gone as low as possible, drive through your heels to stand.

② BB LUNGE

SETS 3 REPS 12 each side TEMPO 1010 REST 60sec

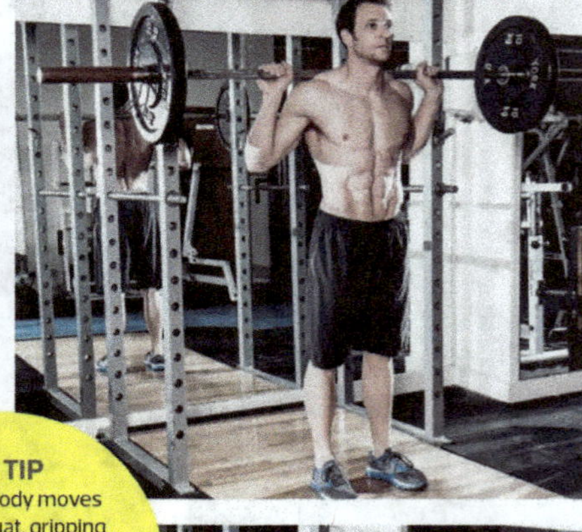

Stand holding the barbell across your traps and take a big lunge forward, allowing your trailing knee to brush the floor. Push off your front foot to return to the start, and repeat on the other side.

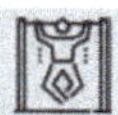

WORKOUT 2

③ ROMANIAN DEADLIFT

SETS 3 REPS 12 TEMPO 1110 REST 60sec

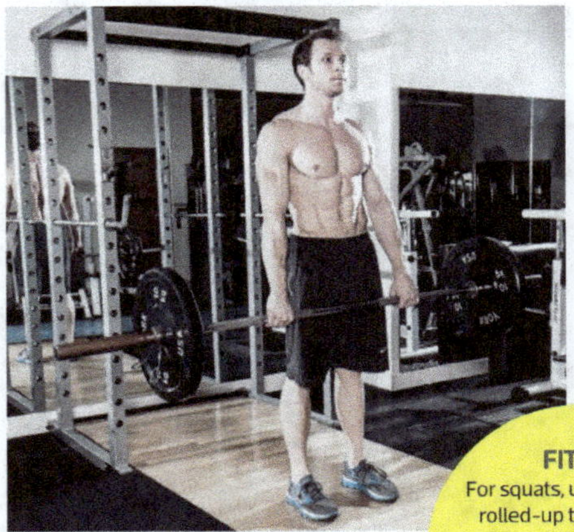

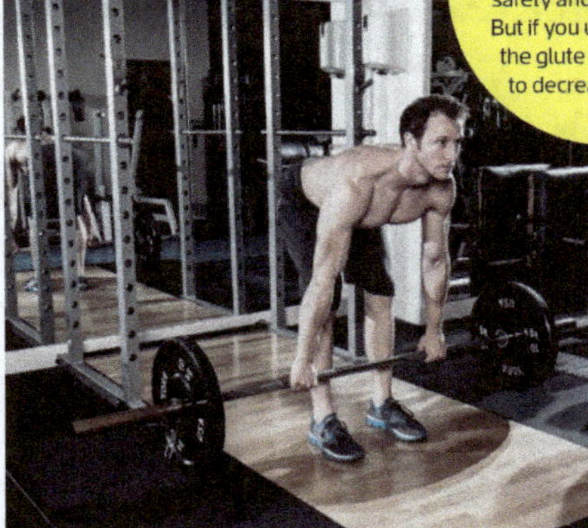

Grab the bar with an overhand grip. Bend your knees slightly, then keep your chest up, shoulders back and maintain a neutral arch in your lower back as you push your hips back. Go as far as you can while keeping the bar close to your body.

④ GLUTE BRIDGE

SETS 3 REPS 12 TEMPO 1110 REST 60sec

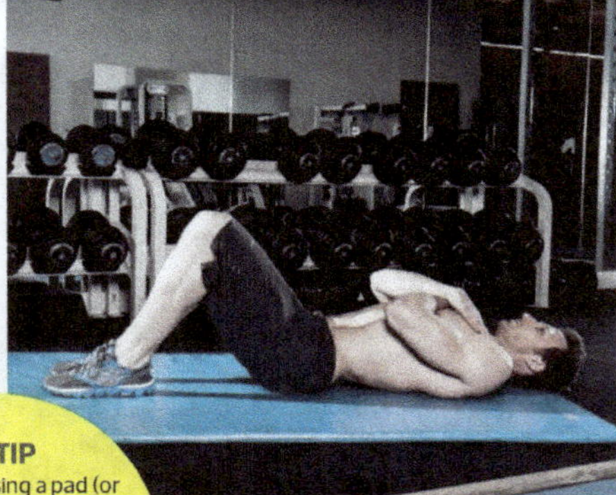

FIT TIP
For squats, using a pad (or rolled-up towel) on the bar can compromise your safety and lifting position. But if you use a barbell for the glute bridge, it's fine to decrease soreness.

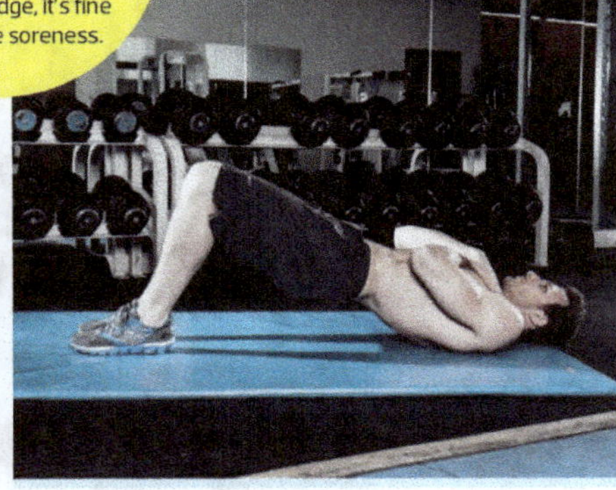

Lie on the floor with your feet close to your glutes. Drive through your heels to raise your hips, tense your glutes at the top of the move, then lower under control. If it's too easy, add a weight plate or barbell.

⑤ BB ROLL-OUT

SETS 3 REPS 12 TEMPO 1111 REST 60sec

Get on your knees with your arms extended and your hands holding a barbell with a shoulder-width grip. Slowly roll the barbell away from your body, keeping your core braced. Go as low as possible, then pull the bar back in.

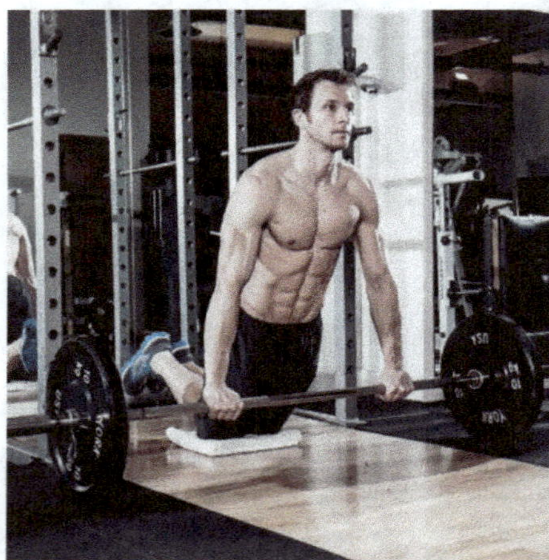

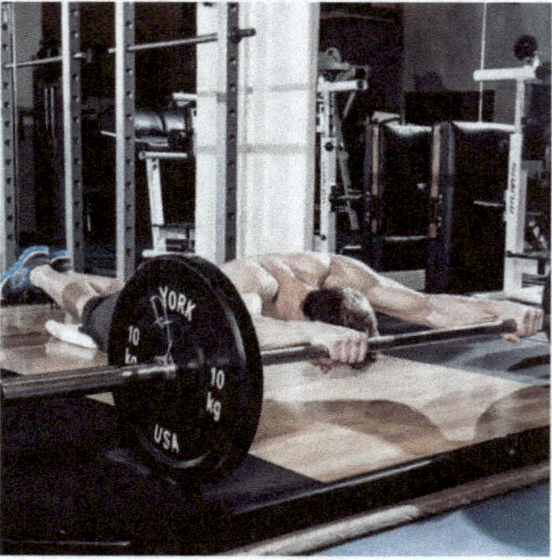

⑥ PLANK

SETS 3 TIME 45sec REST 60sec

Get into a plank position with your forearms on the floor and hands clasped in front of you, then brace your abs and glutes to keep your body in a straight line. Hold that position.

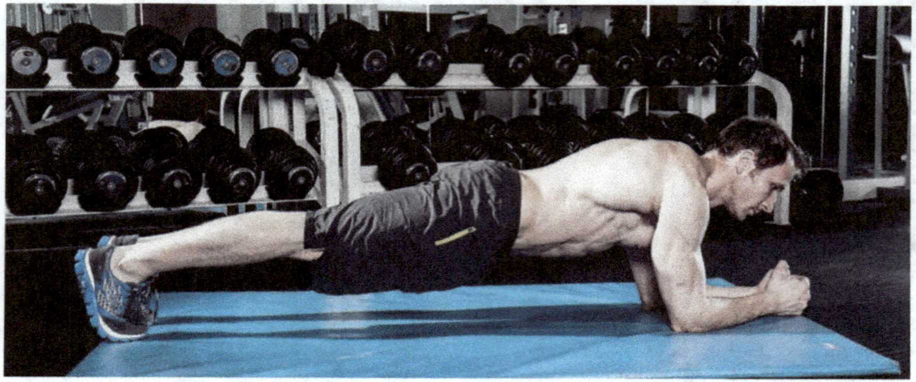

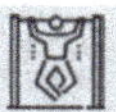

WORKOUT 3

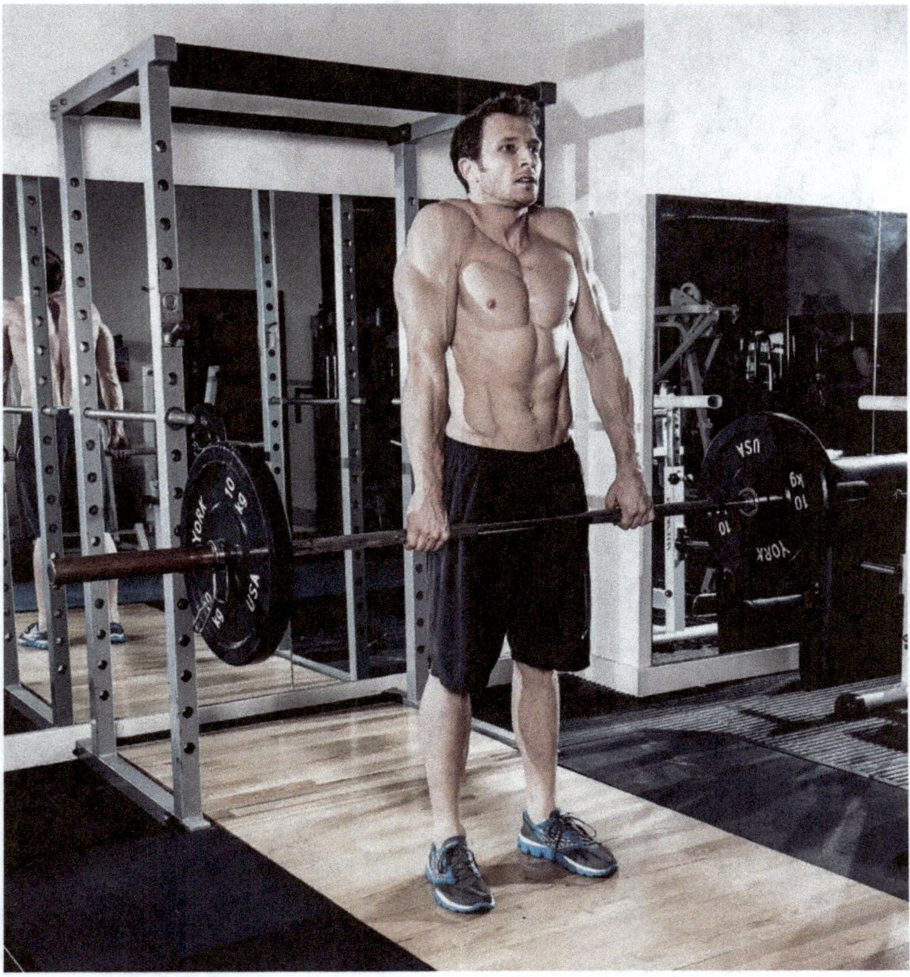

① INCLINE BENCH PRESS

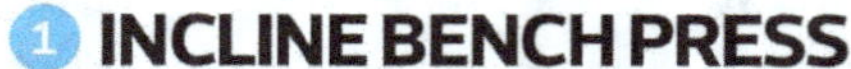

SETS 3 **REPS** 12 **TEMPO** 1010 **REST** 60sec

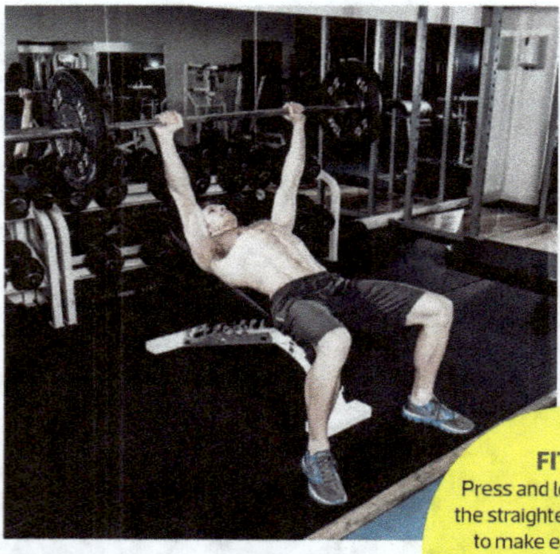

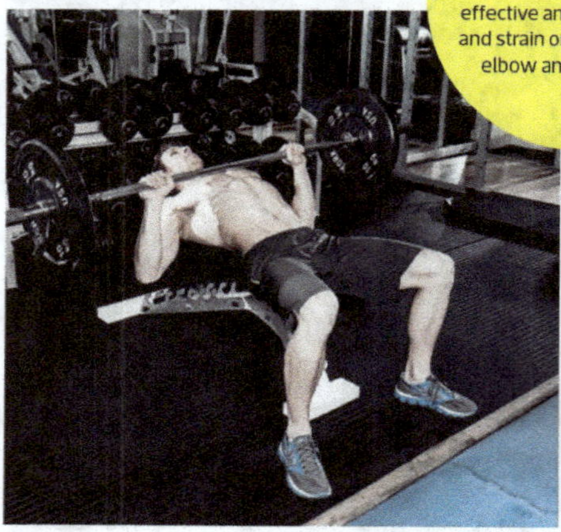

② UNDERHAND ROW

SETS 3 **REPS** 12 **TEMPO** 1110 **REST** 60sec

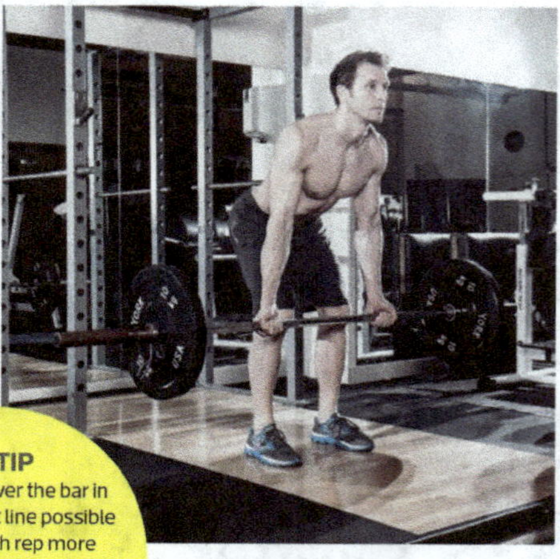

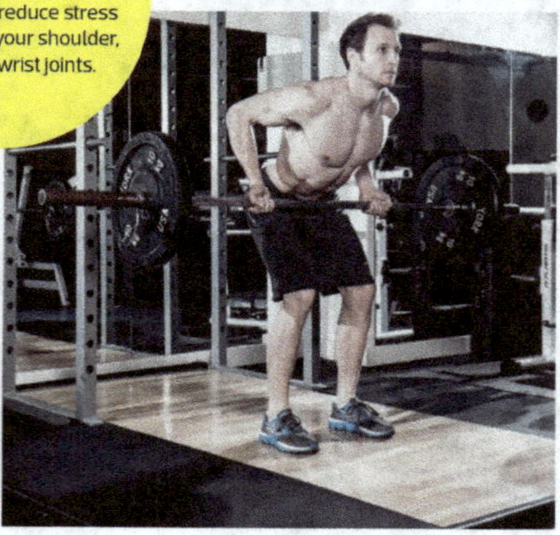

FIT TIP
Press and lower the bar in the straightest line possible to make each rep more effective and reduce stress and strain on your shoulder, elbow and wrist joints.

Lie on an incline bench with your feet on the floor. Hold the bar with an overhand grip with your hands shoulder-width apart. Slowly lower the bar to your chest, then drive it strongly upwards.

Hold a barbell with an underhand grip, so your palms face away. Bend forwards at the hips and pull the bar to your sternum. Pause, and then lower.

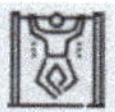

WORKOUT 3

3 PUSH PRESS

SETS 3 **REPS** 12 **TEMPO** 10X0 **REST** 60sec

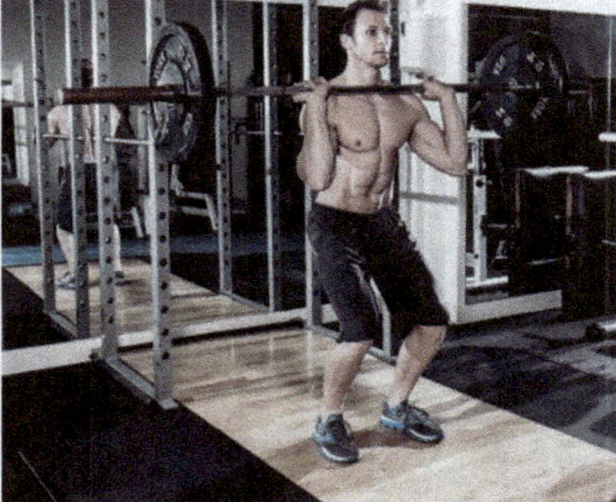

4 EZ-BAR UPRIGHT ROW

SETS 3 **REPS** 12 **TEMPO** 1110 **REST** 60sec

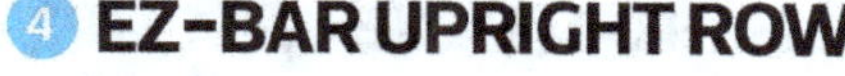

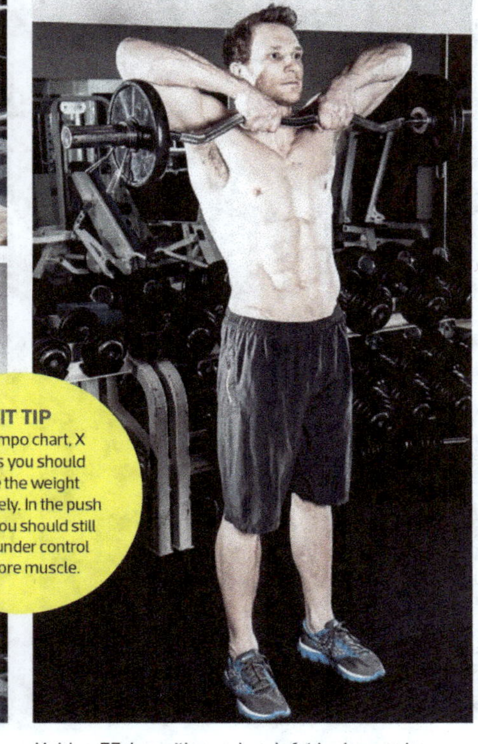

FIT TIP
In a tempo chart, X means you should move the weight explosively. In the push press, you should still lower under control for more muscle.

Hold the bar at shoulder level. Do a quarter-squat to gather momentum, then drive explosively through your heels to help you press the bar overhead. Pause at the top, and lower under control.

Hold an EZ-bar with your hands fairly close, palms facing you. Pull the bar up, bringing your elbows out to the sides, until it's under your chin. Pause, then lower. Don't use momentum – it's bad for your shoulders.

 EZ-BAR REVERSE CURL

SETS 3 REPS 12 TEMPO 1110 REST 60sec

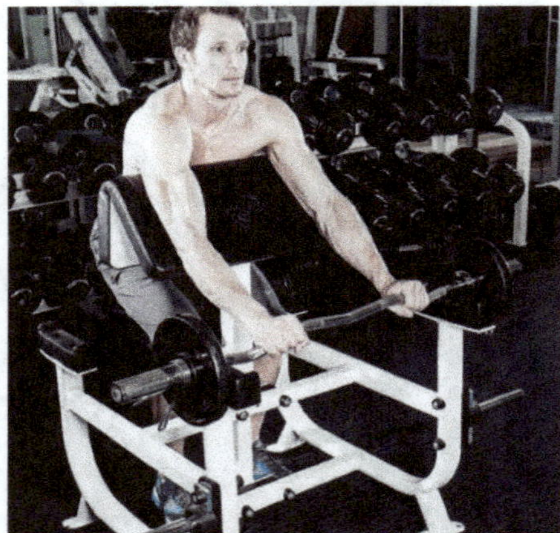

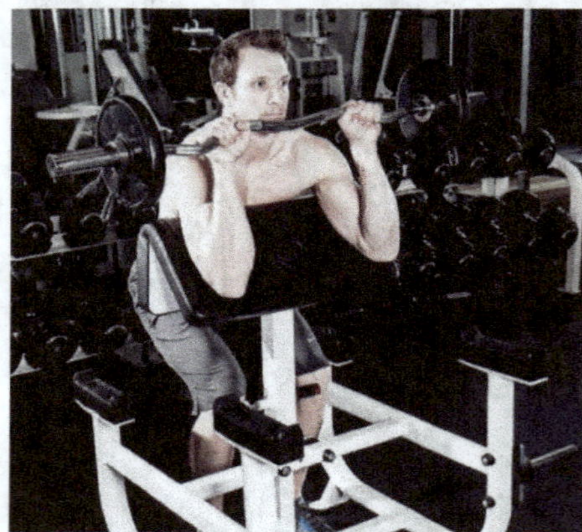

Sit at a preacher bench holding an EZ-bar with your palms down. Curl it up towards your chin, squeeze your biceps at the top, then lower it under control. Reverse curls are harder than normal curls, so you might need to use a lighter weight.

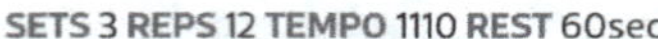 BB SHRUG

SETS 3 REPS 12 TEMPO 1110 REST 60sec

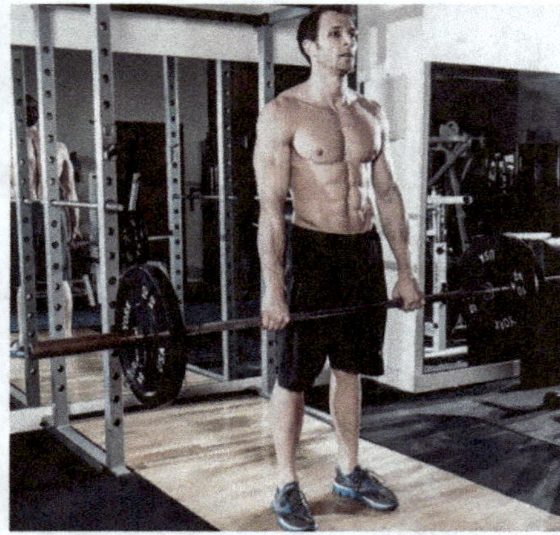

Hold a heavy barbell with an overhand grip and 'shrug' your shoulders directly upwards – not in a circle. Pause, and then lower. If your grip becomes a limiting factor, use chalk or straps.

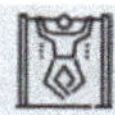

WORKOUT 4

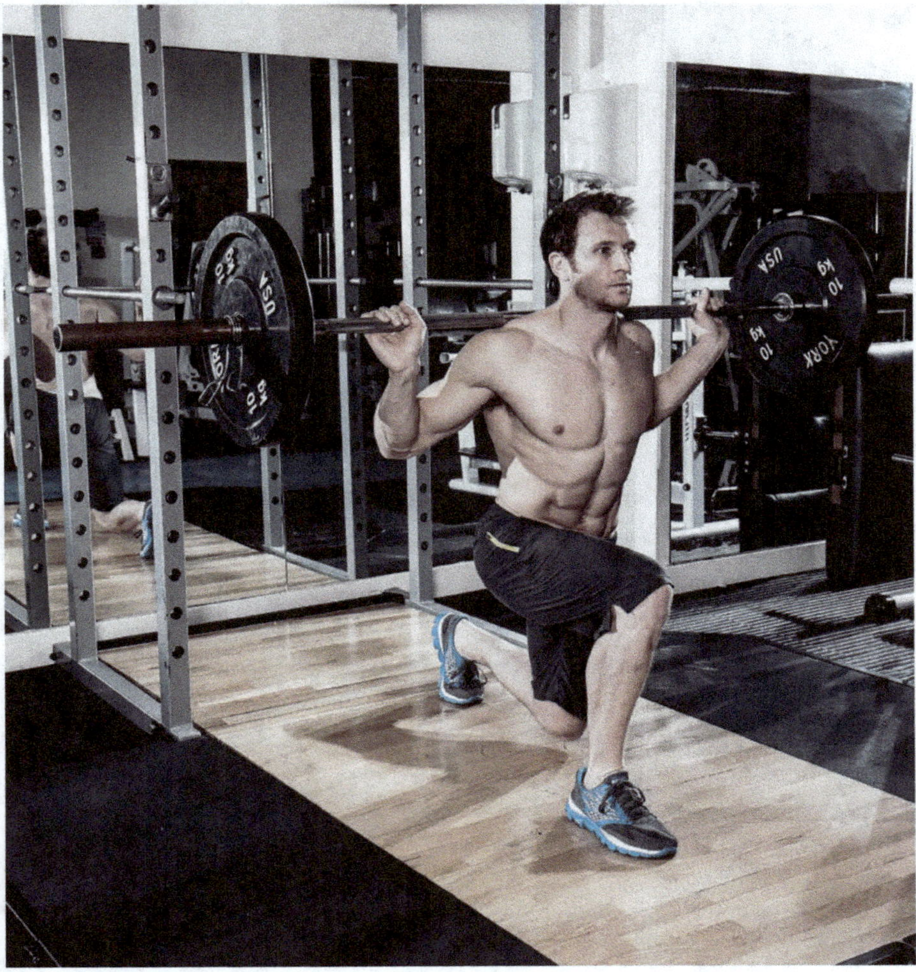

① DEADLIFT

SETS 3 **REPS** 12 **TEMPO** 1010 **REST** 60sec

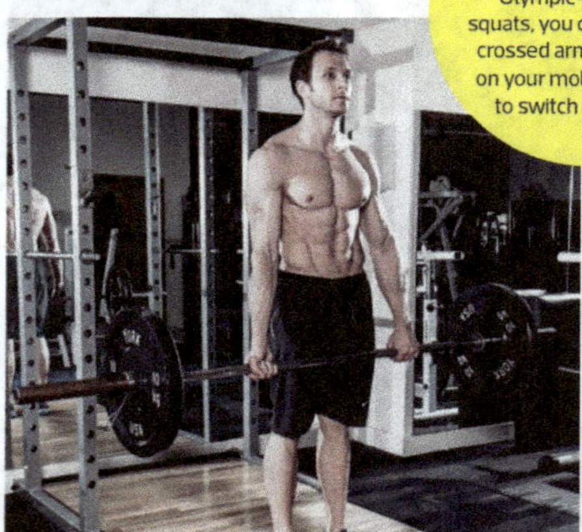

Stand with your toes under the bar, feet hip-width apart. Grab the bar with your arms vertical and just outside your knees. Straighten your back by raising your chest and driving your hips forward, pulling the bar against your shins.

② FRONT SQUAT

SETS 3 **REPS** 12 **TEMPO** 1010 **REST** 60sec

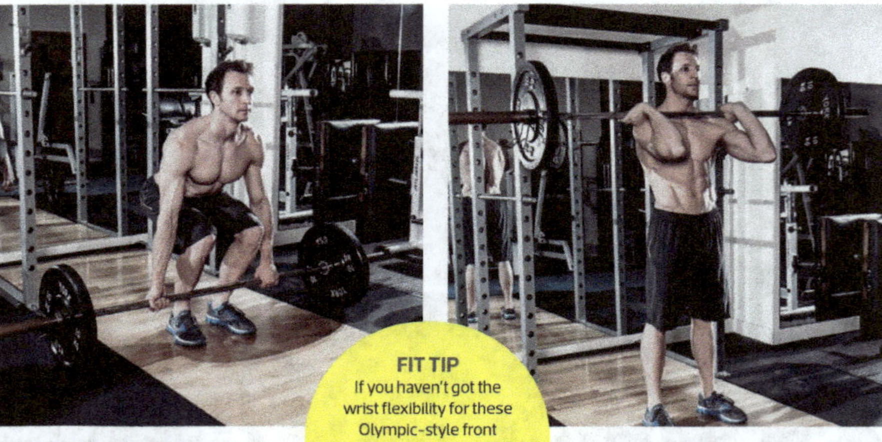

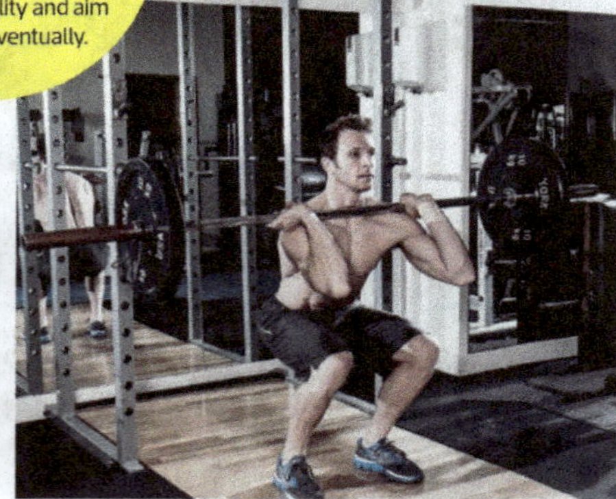

FIT TIP
If you haven't got the wrist flexibility for these Olympic-style front squats, you can squat with crossed arms – but work on your mobility and aim to switch eventually.

Grip the barbell with hands slightly wider than shoulder-width apart and elbows pointing forwards. Unrack the bar, take a deep breath, brace your core and lower under control into a full squat. Drive back up through your midfoot to stand.

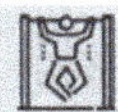

WORKOUT 4

③ BB SPLIT SQUAT

SETS 3 **REPS** 12 each side **TEMPO** 1010 **REST** 60sec

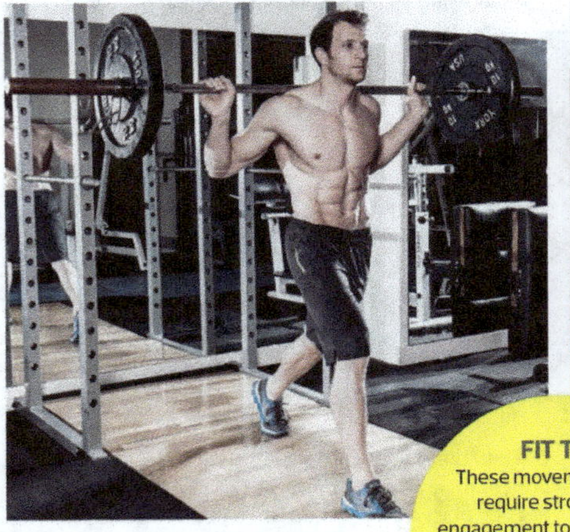

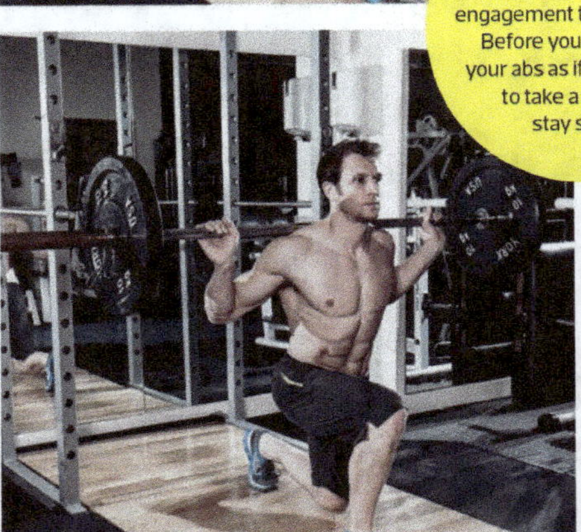

④ GOOD MORNING

SETS 3 **REPS** 12 **TEMPO** 1110 **REST** 60sec

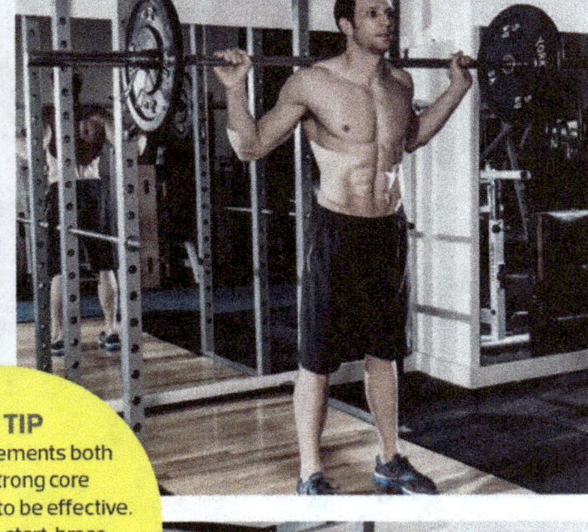

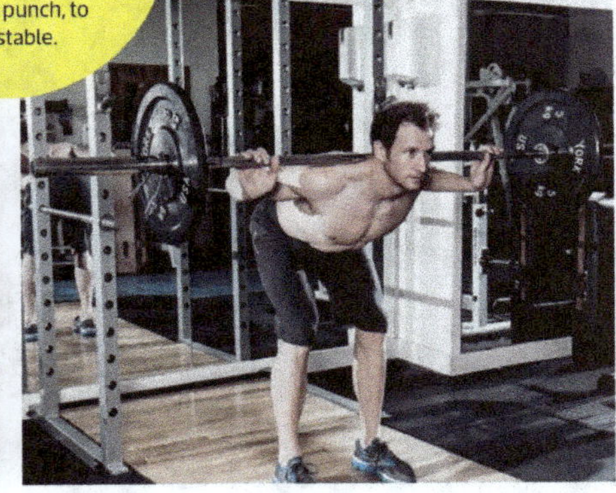

FIT TIP
These movements both require strong core engagement to be effective. Before you start, brace your abs as if you're about to take a punch, to stay stable.

Stand tall with the bar across your upper traps, then take a big step forwards into a lunge position. Bend your knees until your trailing knee brushes the floor, then straighten your rear leg. Alternate sides.

Hold the bar against your traps and bend your knees slightly, then bend forwards at the hips, keeping a neutral spine. Go as close as possible to parallel, then straighten up.

5 SIDE PLANK

SETS 3 **TIME** 45sec each side **REST** 60sec

Get into position on one forearm, with your other hand on your hips – your feet can be staggered for balance, or 'stacked' one on top of the other if you're more advanced. Brace and hold, keeping your body in a straight line.

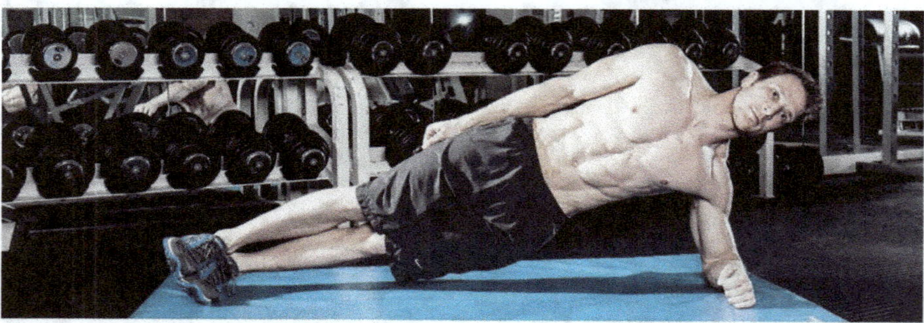

6 SIDE PLANK STAR

SETS 3 **TIME** 45sec each side **REST** 60sec

Get into the side plank position, then raise your upper arm and leg at the same time to increase the tension placed on your core to maintain balance.

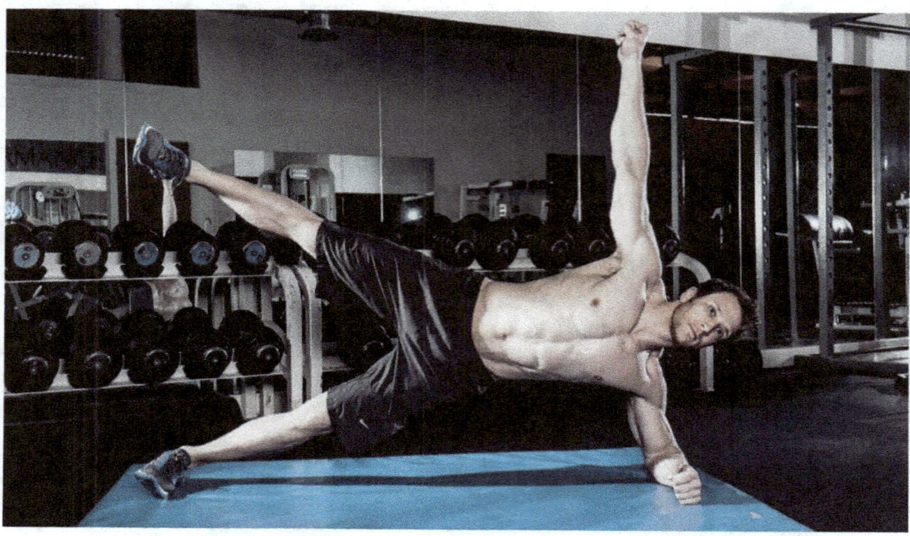

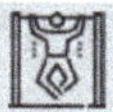

WEEK 4

This final foundation week combines tougher moves with higher volume

WORKOUT 1 **UPPER BODY 1**

EXERCISE	SETS	REPS	TEMPO	REST
1 Bench press	4	10	1010	60SEC
2 Bent-over row	4	10	1110	60SEC
3 Overhead press	4	10	1010	60SEC
4 Lying dumbbell pull-over	4	10	1110	60SEC
5 EZ-bar biceps curl	4	10	1110	60SEC
6 Lying EZ-bar triceps extension	4	10	1010	60SEC

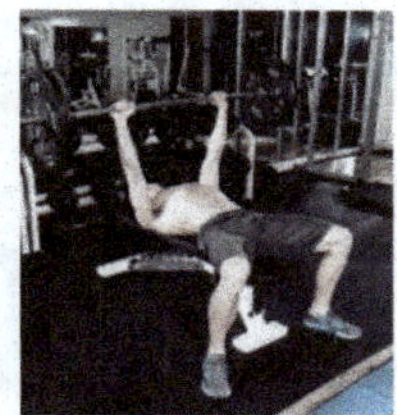

WORKOUT 2 **LOWER BODY 1**

EXERCISE	SETS	REPS/TIME	TEMPO	REST
1 Squat	4	10	1010	60SEC
2 Barbell lunge	4	10 EACH SIDE	1010	60SEC
3 Romanian deadlift	4	10	1110	60SEC
4 Glute bridge	4	10	1110	60SEC
5 Barbell roll-out	4	10	1111	60SEC
6 Plank	4	45SEC	N/A	60SEC

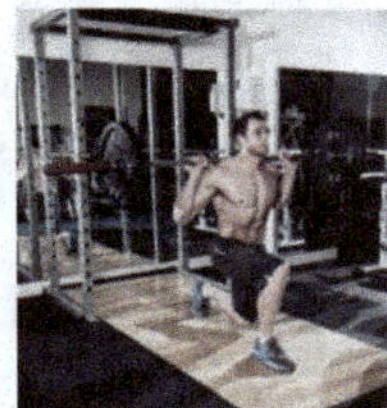

WORKOUT 3 **UPPER BODY 2**

EXERCISE	SETS	REPS	TEMPO	REST
1 Incline bench press	4	10	1010	60SEC
2 Underhand bent-over row	4	10	1110	60SEC
3 Push press	4	10	1010	60SEC
4 EZ-bar upright row	4	10	1110	60SEC
5 EZ-bar reverse curl	4	10	1110	60SEC
6 Barbell shrug	4	10	1110	60SEC

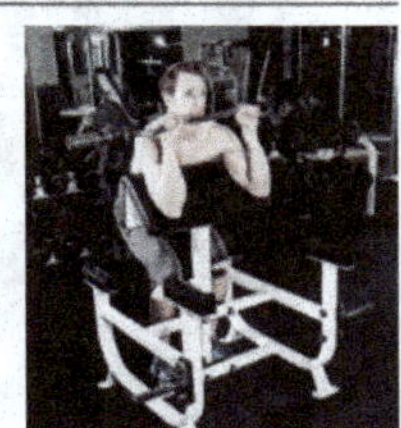

WORKOUT 4 **LOWER BODY 2**

EXERCISE	SETS	REPS/TIME	TEMPO	REST
1 Deadlift	4	10	1010	60SEC
2 Front squat	4	10	1010	60SEC
3 Barbell split squat	4	10 EACH SIDE	1010	60SEC
4 Good morning	4	10	1110	60SEC
5 Side plank	4	45SEC EACH SIDE	N/A	60SEC
6 Side plank star	4	45SEC EACH SIDE	N/A	60SEC

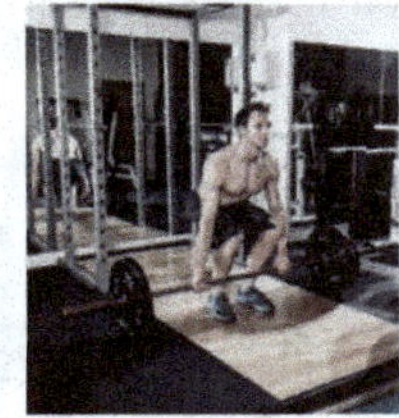

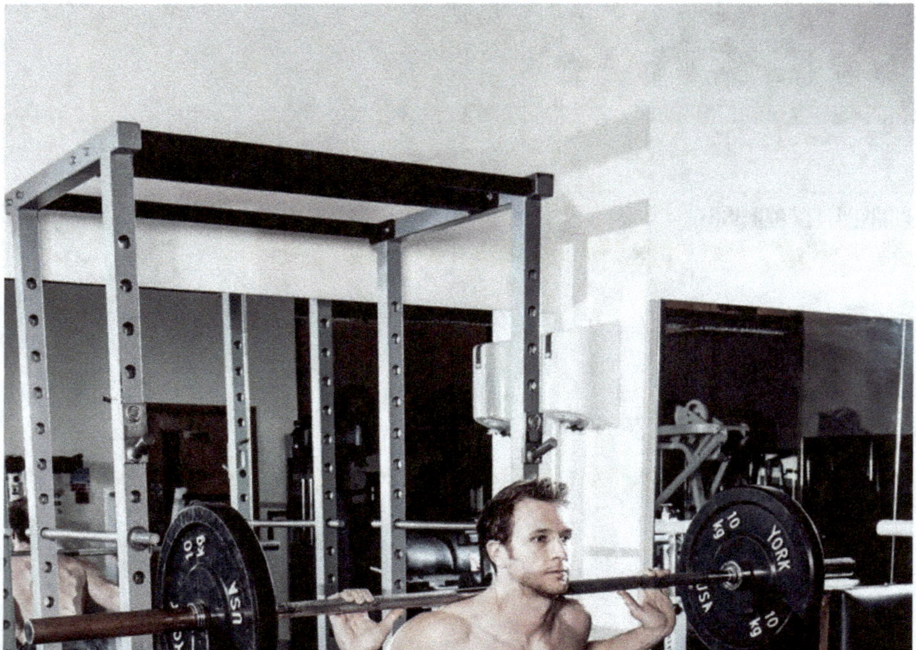

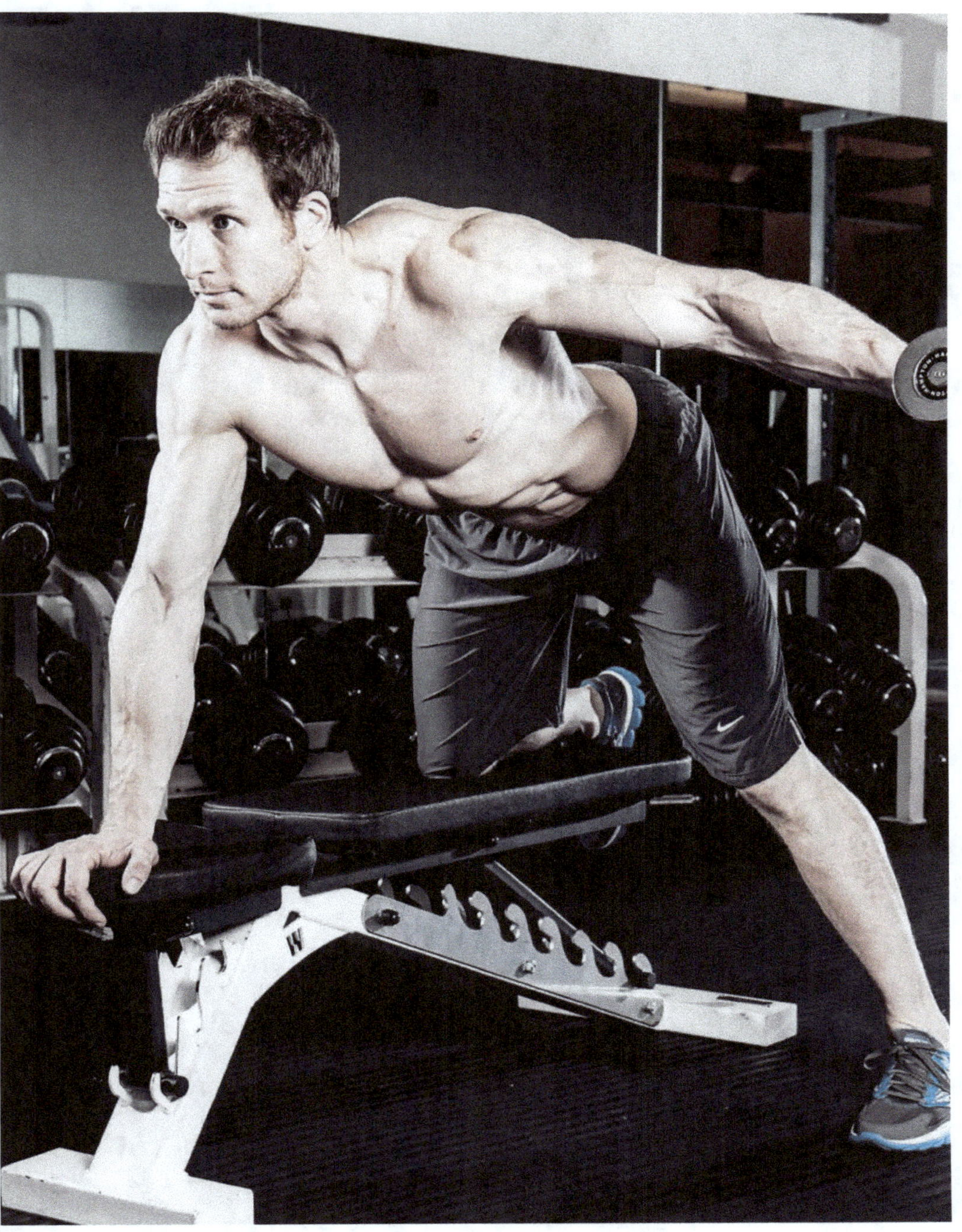

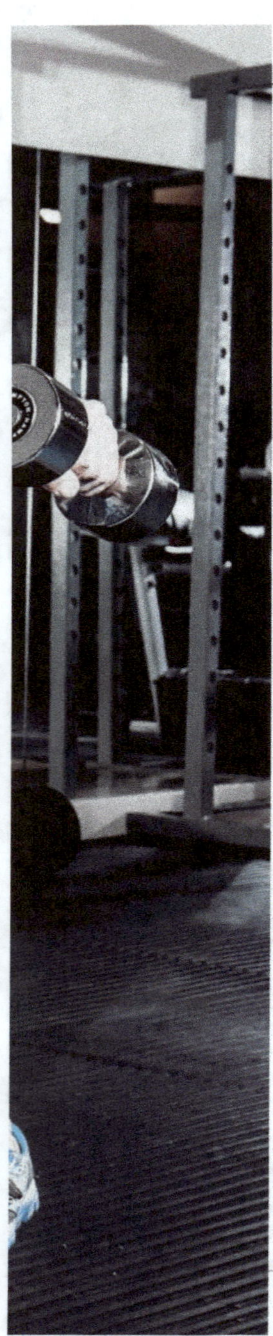

GET STRONGER – FASTER

The second phase of your plan uses supersets and paired movements to help you make quick gains

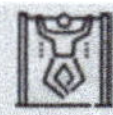

STRENGTH BEFORE MUSCLE

In this phase of your programme, things get tougher. You'll shift from an upper-lower body focus to a more traditional bodybuilding training split, hitting each body part once a week: one workout each for chest and triceps, back and biceps, legs, and shoulders and core. This means more sets for each muscle per workout, which means you'll need to grit your teeth and push through. But the good news is you'll also be hitting your muscles from multiple angles – crucial in the case of body parts such as the shoulder, where maximum size means hitting all three heads of the muscle (front, back and side). You'll still do the first two moves in each workout as standalone movements, but the other four movements in each session are done as supersets, which means you'll pair movements and alternate sets between them. So where the exercises are marked A and B, you do one set of move A, rest as indicated, then one set of B, then rest, and continue till you complete all the reps. This technique enables you to hit a muscle group harder and from different angles in the same session, helping you to build strength and kick-starting the hypertrophy process.

Finally, by including more isolation-heavy movements – EZ-bar curls, for example – you'll also hit individual muscles harder during this phase. It's not easy, but give every workout all you've got, and you'll grow fast.

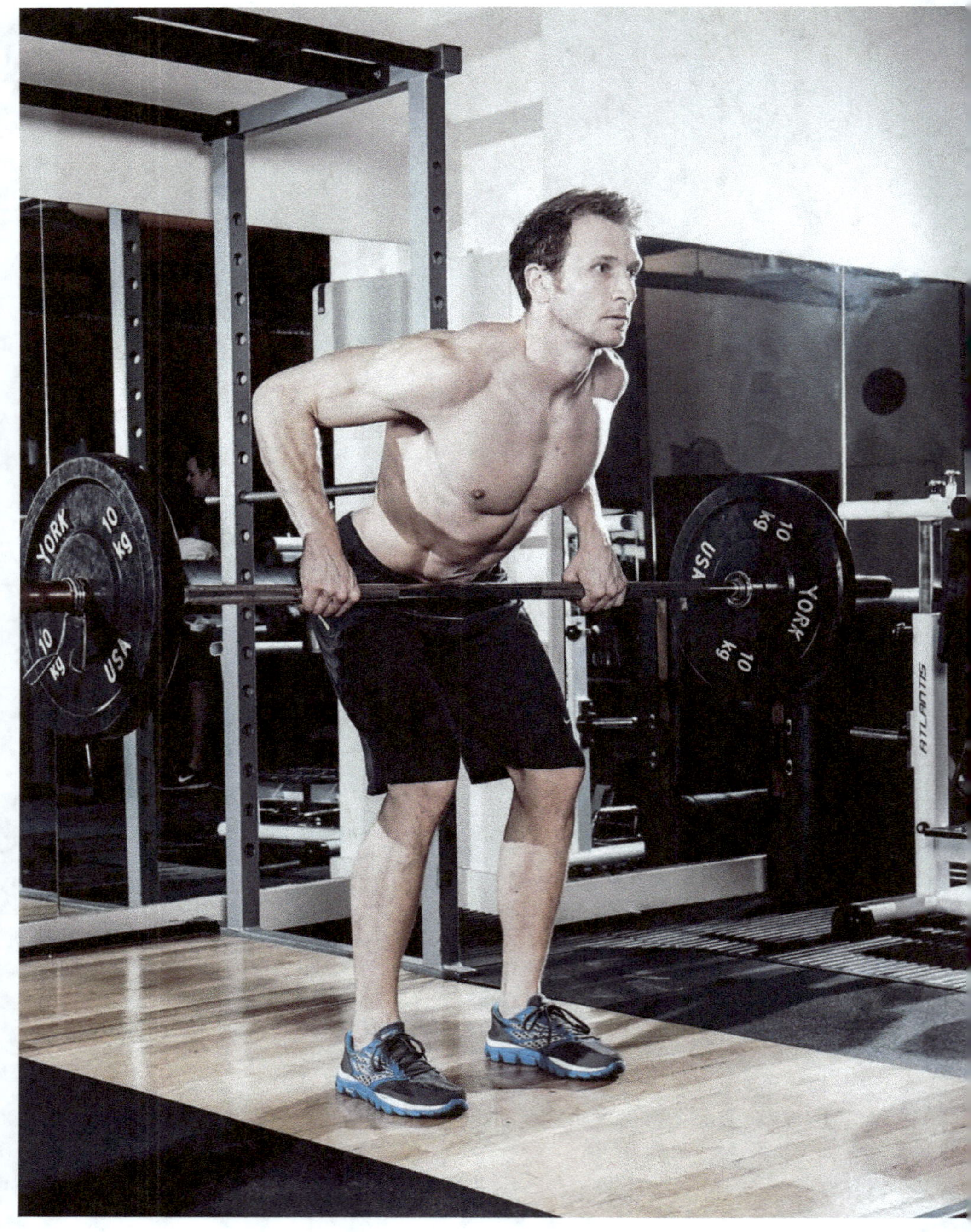

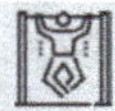

WEEK 1 WORKOUT 1

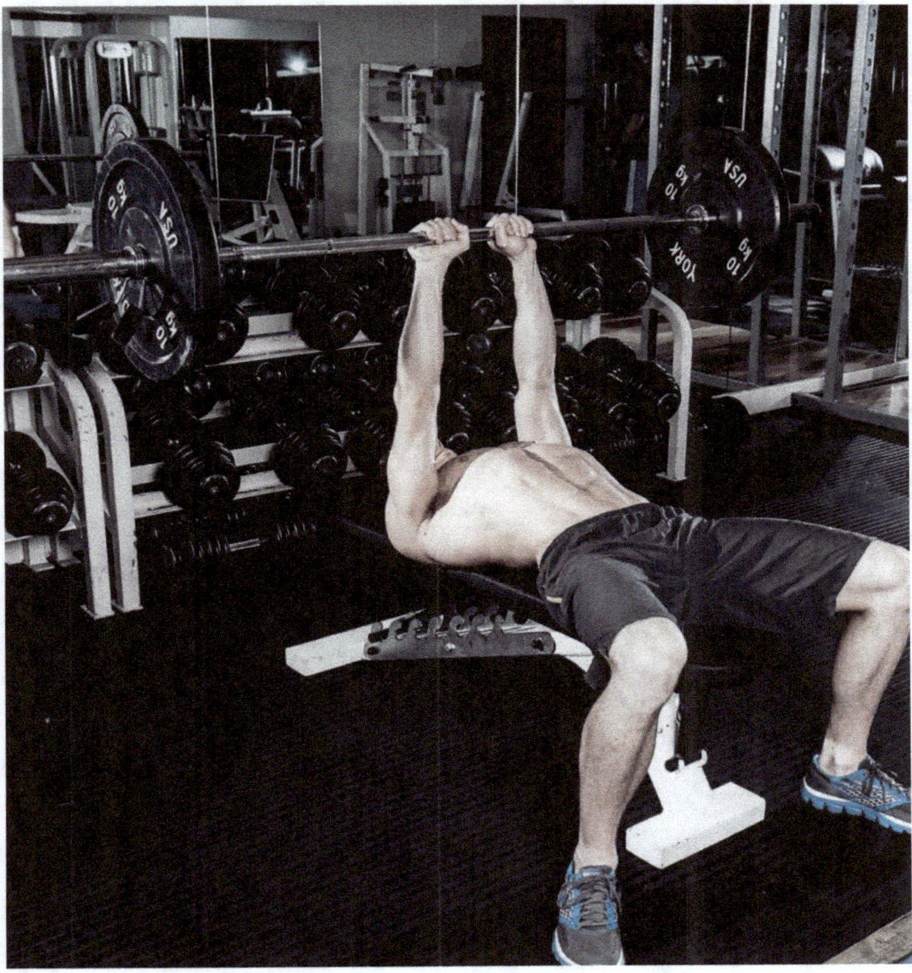

① BENCH PRESS

SETS 5 REPS 10 TEMPO 1010 REST 90sec

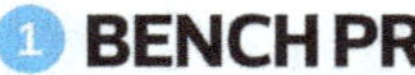

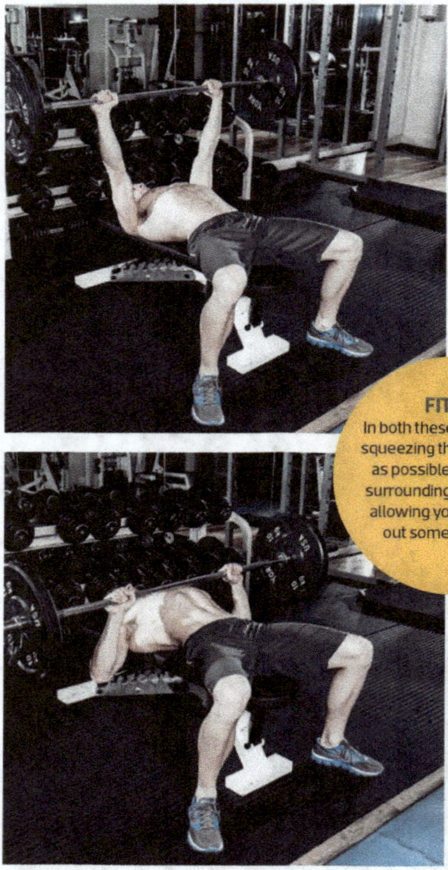

Lie on the bench with your feet on the floor. Hold the bar with your hands shoulder-width apart. Slowly lower the bar to your chest. Drive your feet hard into the floor and push the bar back strongly to the start position.

② TRICEPS DIP

SETS 5 REPS 10 TEMPO 1010 REST 90sec

FIT TIP
In both these movements, squeezing the bars as hard as possible will help the surrounding muscles fire, allowing you to squeeze out some extra reps.

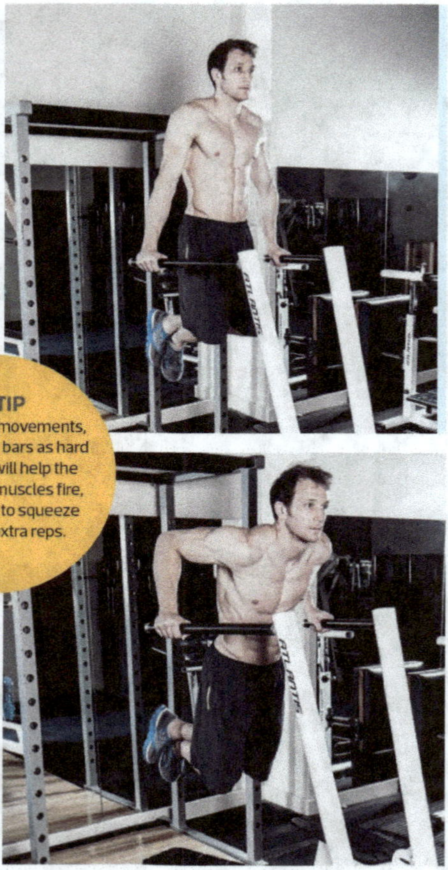

Grip a set of dip bars with your hands roughly shoulder-width apart, arms straight. Lower yourself until your upper arms are parallel to the floor, keeping your chest upright to hit your triceps. Press back up.

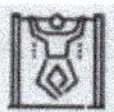

WORKOUT 1

3 A INCLINE DB BENCH PRESS

SETS 3 REPS 8 TEMPO 1010 REST 60sec

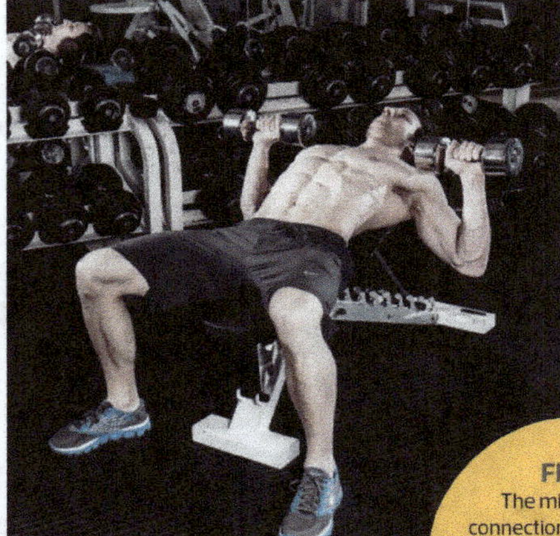

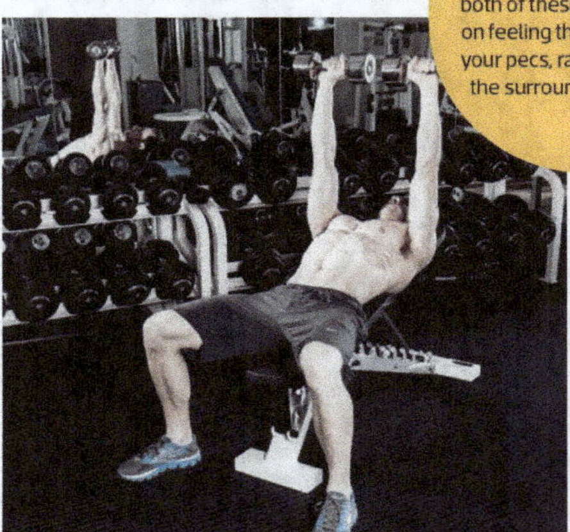

Lie on a bench set at a 30° angle holding a dumbbell in each hand. Keep your feet flat on the floor and your back against the bench. Press the weights straight up, without locking out at the top, then lower.

3 B INCLINE DB FLYE

SETS 3 REPS 8 TEMPO 1010 REST 60sec

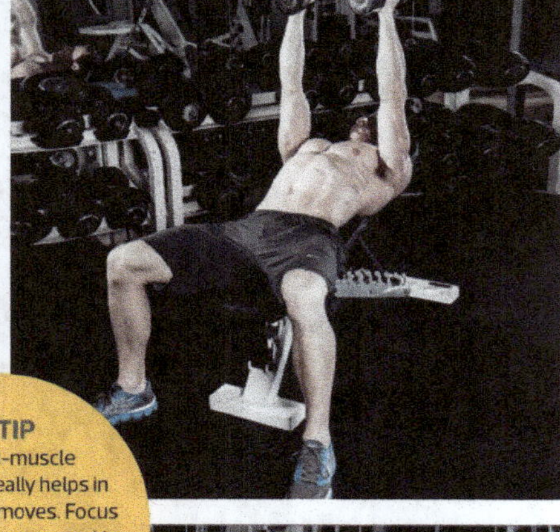

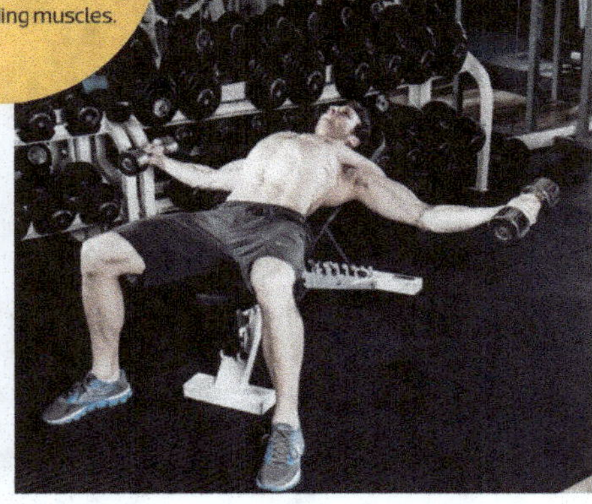

Lie on a bench set at an incline, holding dumbbells above you, palms facing in. Lower your arms out to the sides with your elbows slightly bent, until you feel a stretch in your chest, then bring them together.

FIT TIP
The mind-muscle connection really helps in both of these moves. Focus on feeling the movement in your pecs, rather than using the surrounding muscles.

4 A CLOSE-GRIP BENCH PRESS

SETS 3 REPS 8 TEMPO 1010 REST 60sec

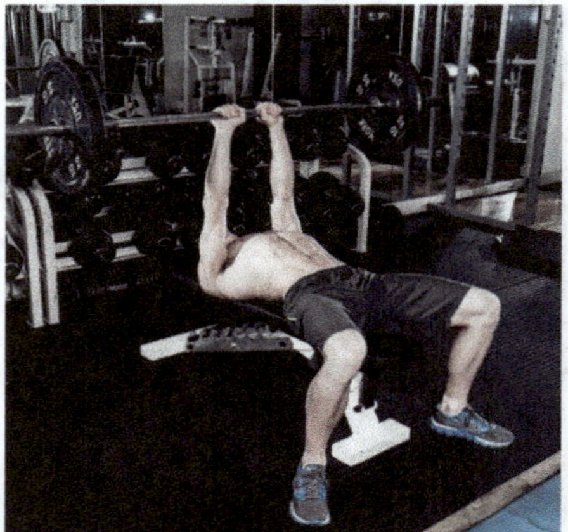

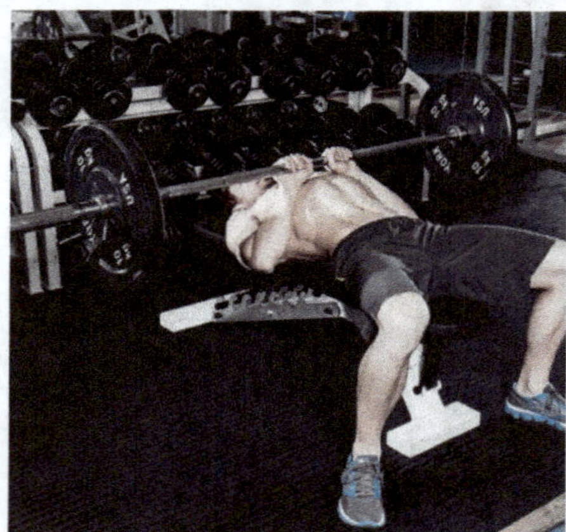

Lie on a bench and grip a barbell with your hands just narrower than shoulder-width apart. Lower the barbell to your chest, keeping your elbows close to your sides. Pause, and then press back up.

4 B LYING TRICEPS EXTENSION

SETS 3 REPS 8 TEMPO 1010 REST 60sec

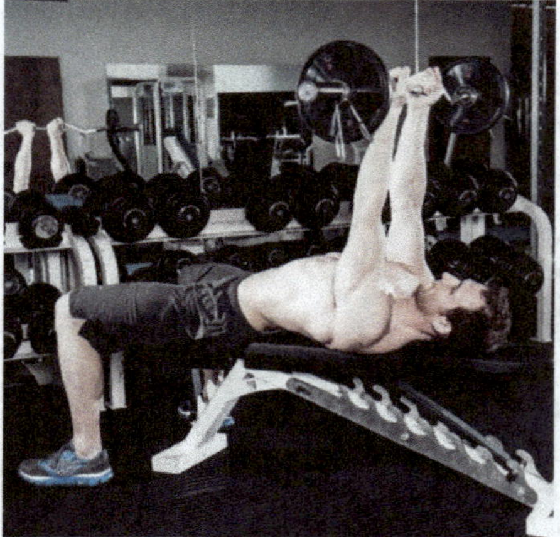

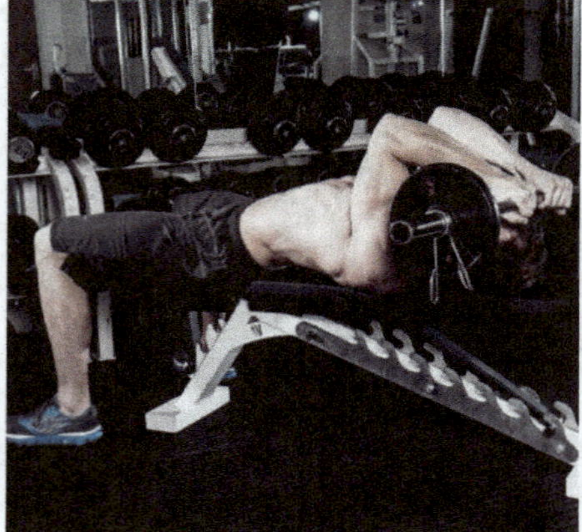

Lie on a bench with an EZ-bar held overhead, arms straight. Lower the bar towards your forehead by bending your arms. Pause, then use your triceps to raise the weight back to the start.

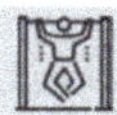

WORKOUT 2

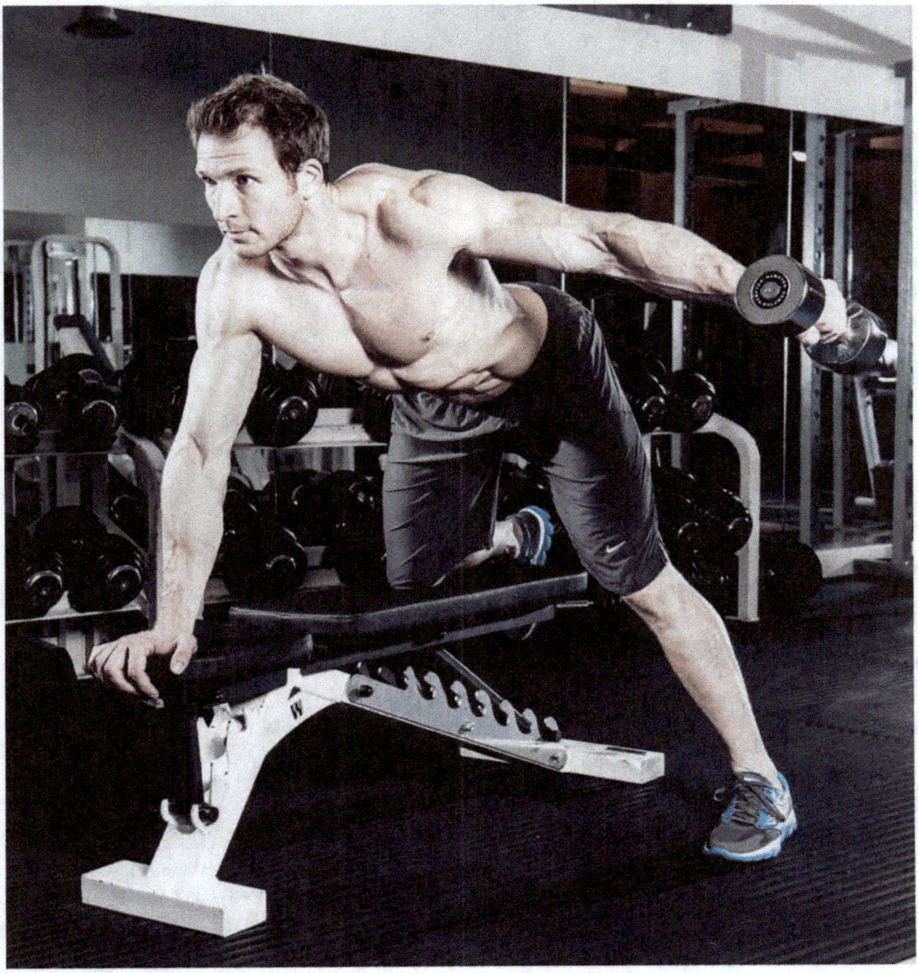

① BENT-OVER ROW

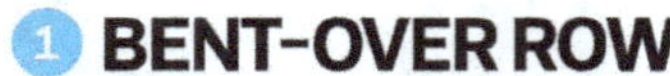

SETS 5 **REPS** 10 **TEMPO** 1010 **REST** 90sec

② CHIN-UP

SETS 5 **REPS** 6–10 **TEMPO** 1010 **REST** 90sec

FIT TIP
Aim to go to technical failure on the chin-ups. That means complete as many reps as possible, but don't crank out sloppy reps or you won't get the full effect.

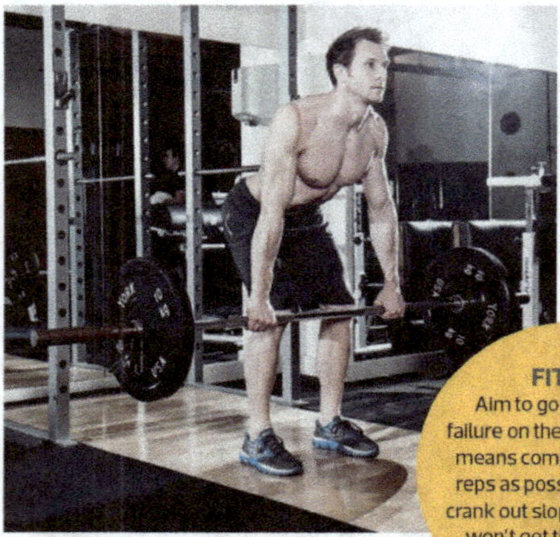

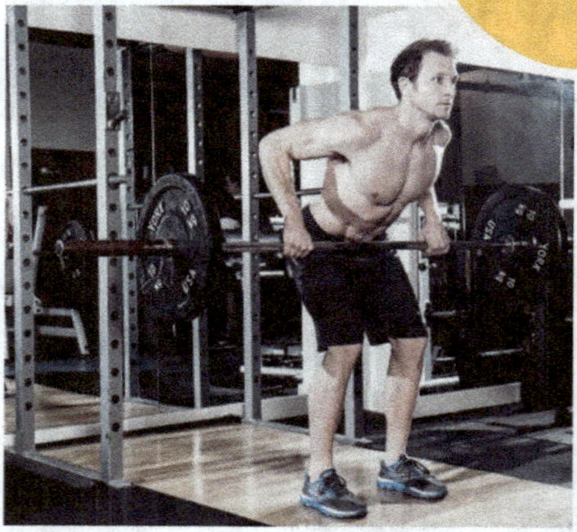

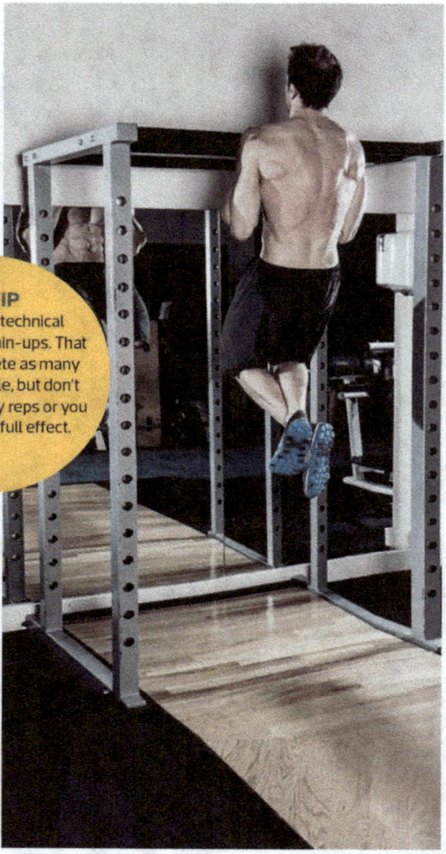

Bend your knees slightly and lean forwards with your hands just wider than shoulder-width apart on the bar. Pull the bar up to your lower sternum, focusing on pulling your elbows behind you, then lower under control.

Hang from a bar with your palms facing towards you, shoulder blades retracted. Pull yourself up until your chin is above the bar, pause, then lower until your arms are straight again.

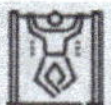

WORKOUT 2

  ## DB ONE-ARM ROW

SETS 3 **REPS** 8 each side **TEMPO** 1010 **REST** 60sec

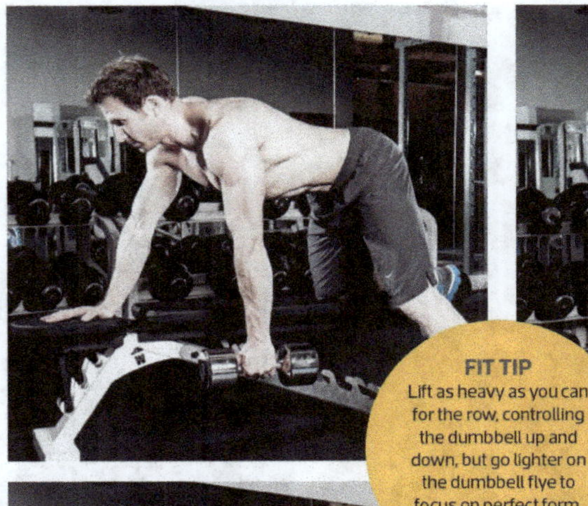

FIT TIP
Lift as heavy as you can for the row, controlling the dumbbell up and down, but go lighter on the dumbbell flye to focus on perfect form.

Place one knee on a bench, supporting your torso with a straight arm, holding a dumbbell in the other hand. With your foot flat and core braced, row the weight up, leading with your elbow, then lower. Do all the reps on one side, then switch.

DB ONE-ARM BENT FLYE

SETS 3 **REPS** 8 each side **TEMPO** 1010 **REST** 60sec

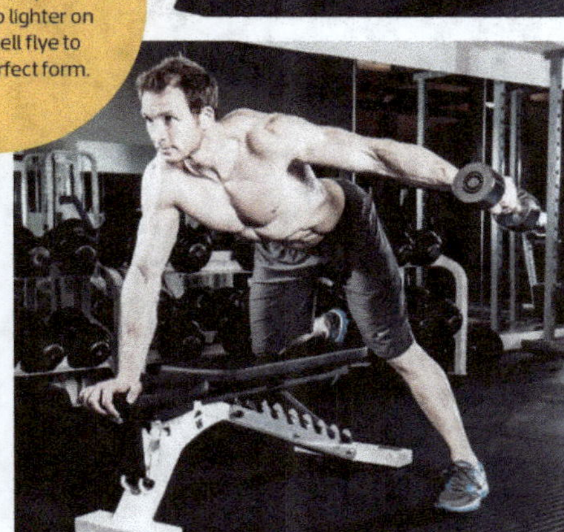

Place one knee on a bench, supporting your torso with a straight arm, holding a dumbbell in the other hand. With your foot flat and core braced, raise the weight to shoulder height, then lower slowly. Do all the reps on one side, then switch.

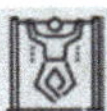

4 A EZ-BAR BICEPS CURL

SETS 3 REPS 8 TEMPO 1010 REST 60sec

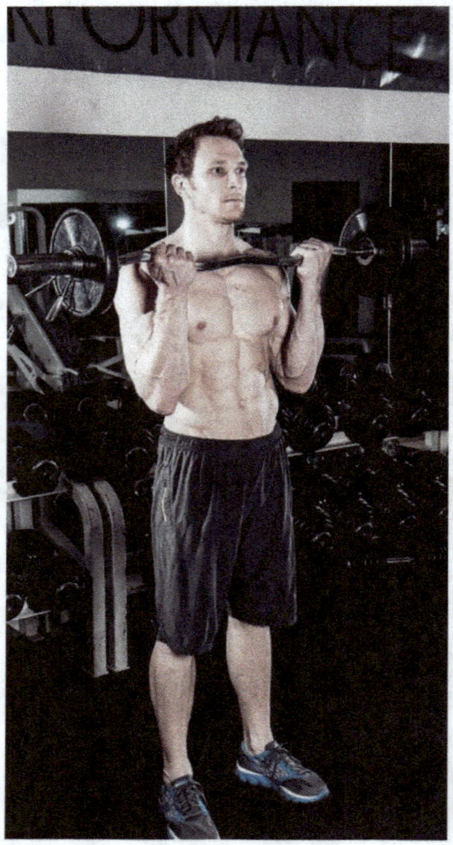

Using an EZ-bar reduces stress on your elbows. Stand straight and curl the bar upwards. Squeeze your biceps at the top of the movement and your triceps at the bottom.

4 B EZ-BAR REVERSE CURL

SETS 3 REPS 8 TEMPO 1010 REST 60sec

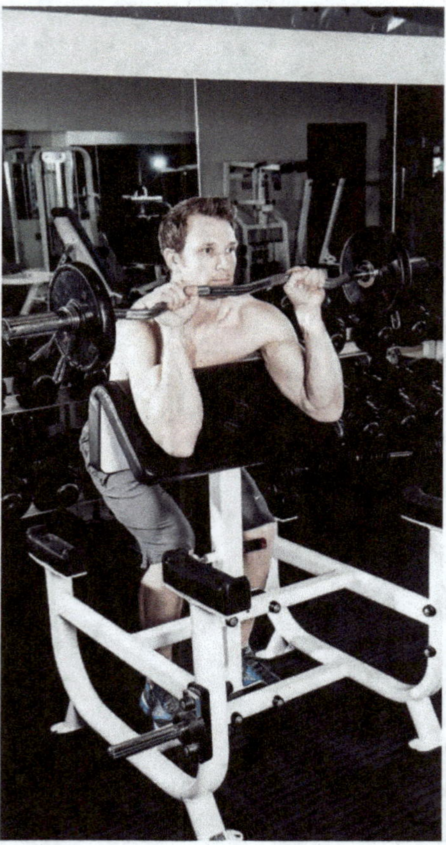

Sit at a preacher bench holding an EZ-bar with your palms down. Curl it up towards your chin, squeeze your biceps at the top, then lower it under control. Reverse curls are harder than normal curls, so you might need to use a lighter weight.

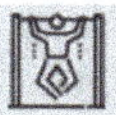

WORKOUT 3

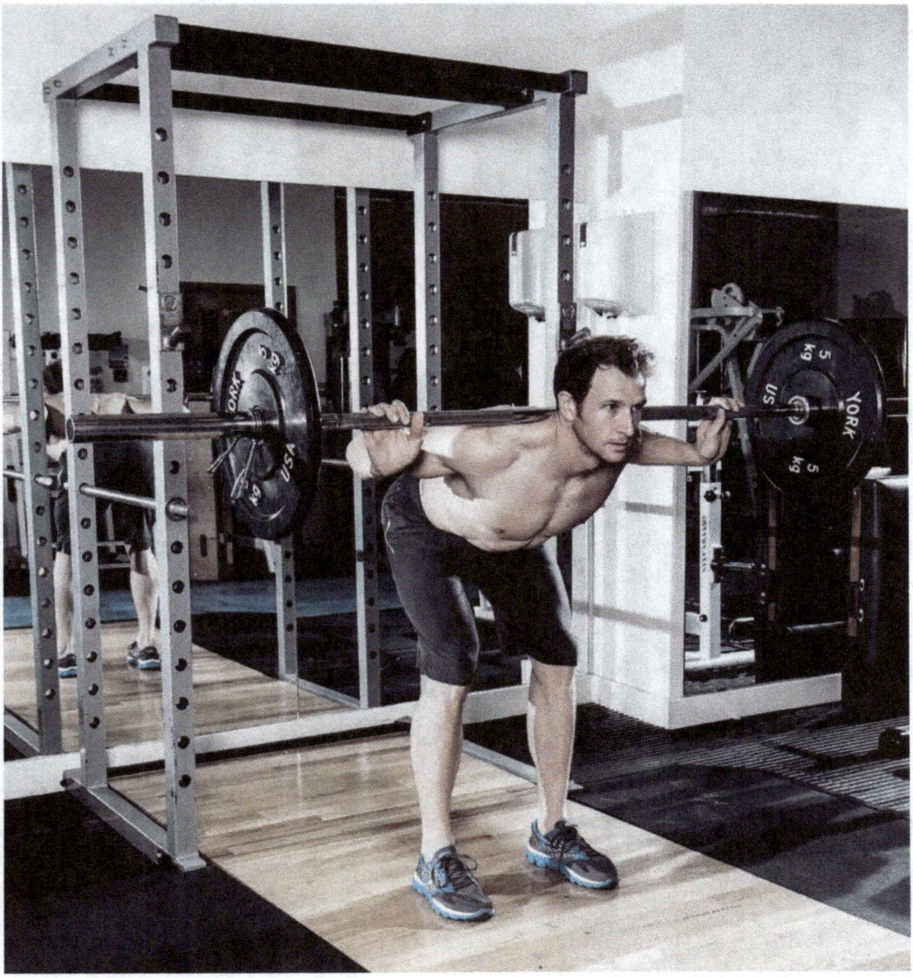

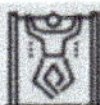

① DEADLIFT

SETS 5 **REPS** 10 **TEMPO** 1010 **REST** 90sec

② BB SQUAT

SETS 5 **REPS** 10 **TEMPO** 1010 **REST** 90sec

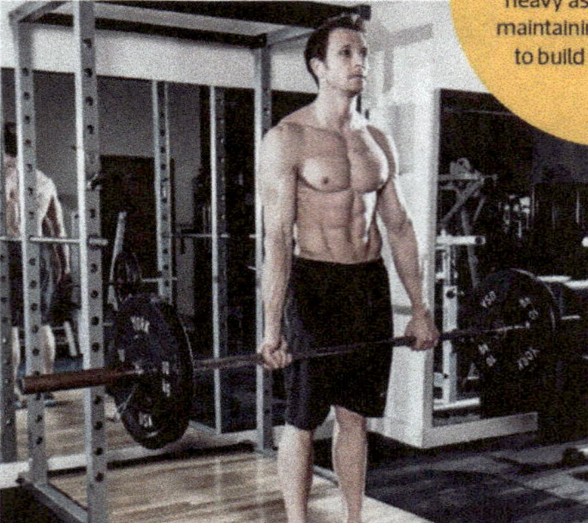

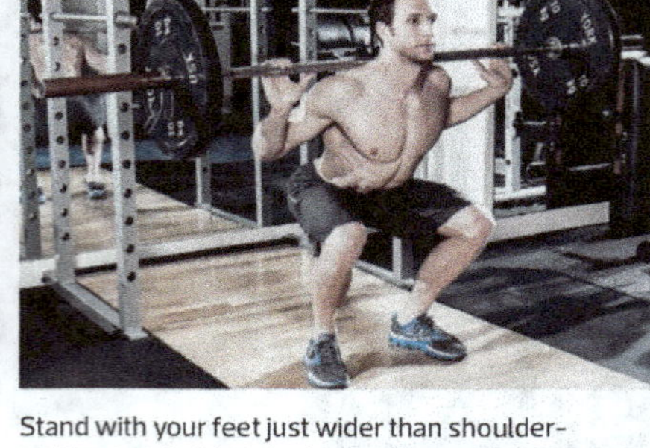

FIT TIP
For these two classic big compound lifts you want to go as heavy as you can while maintaining perfect form to build raw strength.

Stand with your toes under the bar, feet hip-width apart. Grab the bar with your arms vertical and just outside your knees. Straighten your back by raising your chest and driving your hips forward, pulling the bar against your shins.

Stand with your feet just wider than shoulder-width apart, holding the bar on your upper traps. Sit down and back, keeping your chest up and your core engaged. When you've gone as low as possible, drive through your heels to stand.

 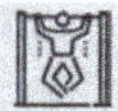

WORKOUT 3

  ## DB LUNGE

SETS 3 REPS 8 each side TEMPO 1010 REST 60sec

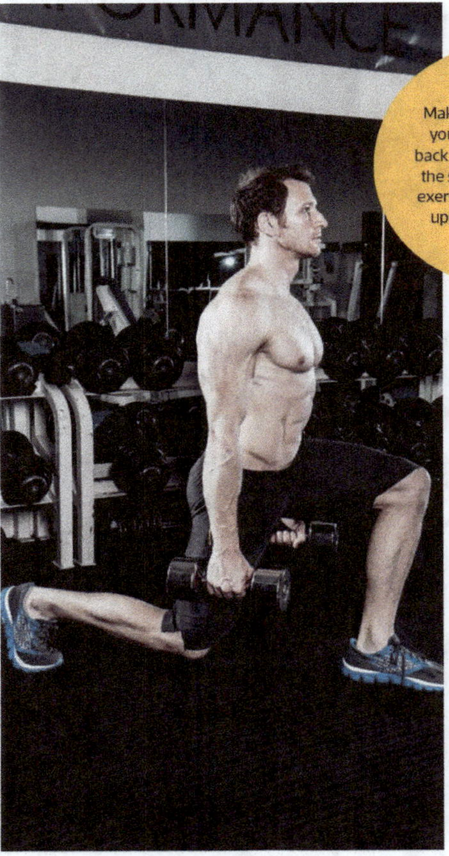

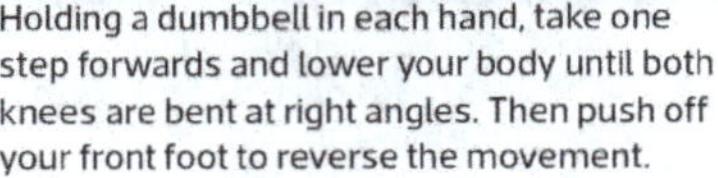

Holding a dumbbell in each hand, take one step forwards and lower your body until both knees are bent at right angles. Then push off your front foot to reverse the movement.

3 B DB ROMANIAN DEADLIFT

SETS 3 REPS 8 TEMPO 1010 REST 60sec

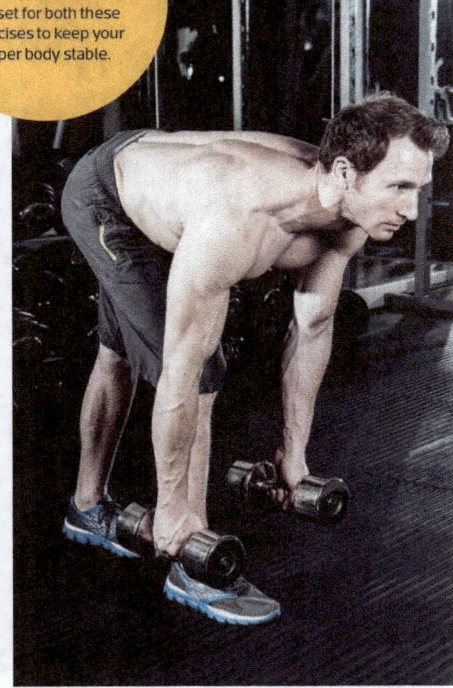

Holding a set of dumbbells and keeping a slight bend in your knees, bend forwards from the hips and lower the dumbbells until you feel a stretch in your hamstrings. Reverse the move back to the start and push your hips forwards.

 # GOOD MORNING

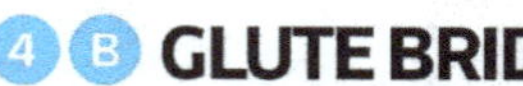 # GLUTE BRIDGE

SETS 3 REPS 8 TEMPO 1010 REST 60sec

SETS 3 REPS 8 TEMPO 1010 REST 60sec

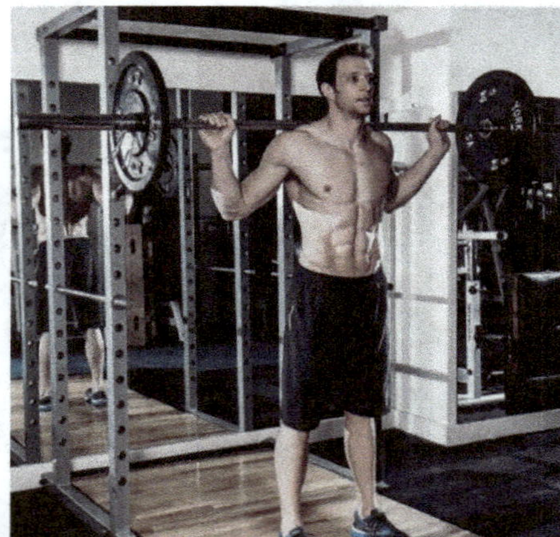

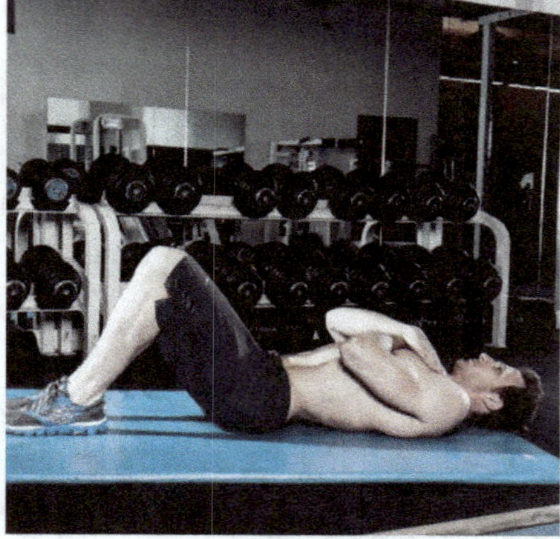

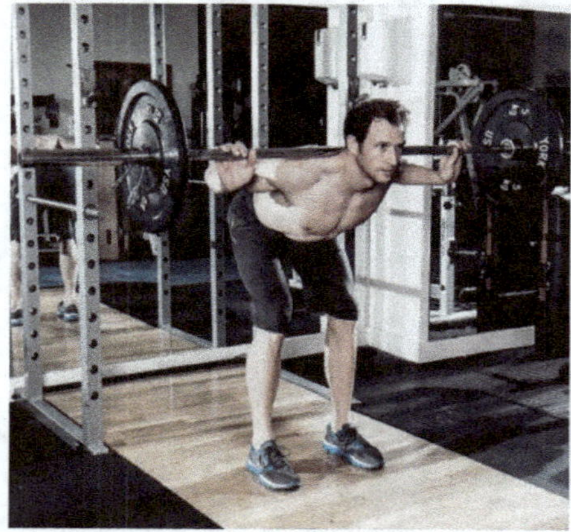

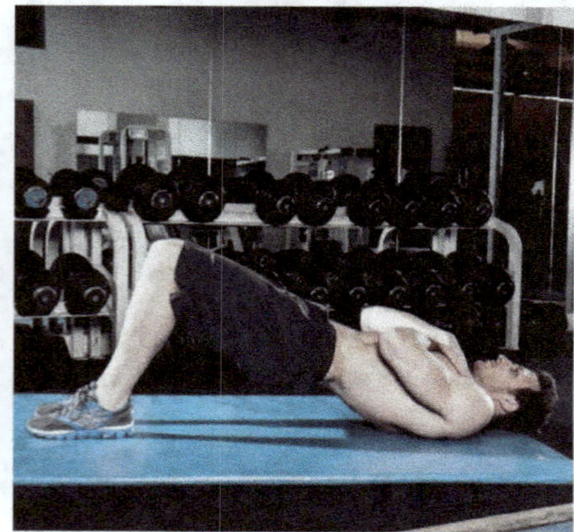

Hold the bar against your traps and bend your knees slightly, then bend forwards at the hips, keeping a neutral spine. Go as close as possible to parallel, then straighten up.

Lie on the floor with your feet close to your glutes. Drive through your heels to raise your hips, tense your glutes at the top of the move, then lower under control. If it's too easy, add a weight plate or barbell.

 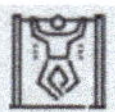

WORKOUT 4

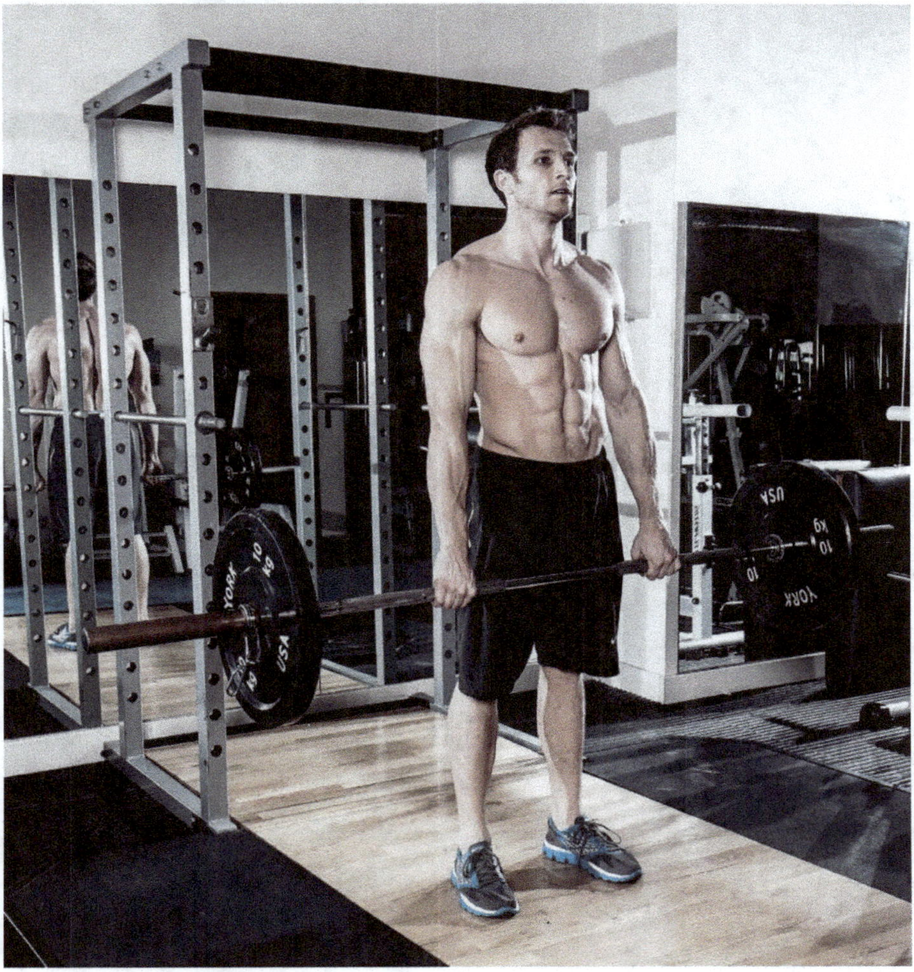

① OVERHEAD PRESS

SETS 5 **REPS** 10 **TEMPO** 1010 **REST** 90sec

② EZ-BAR UPRIGHT ROW

SETS 5 **REPS** 10 **TEMPO** 1010 **REST** 90sec

FIT TIP
In both of these movements, you'll get superior results from using a weight that you can manage with very strict form, rather than relying on leg drive to power through.

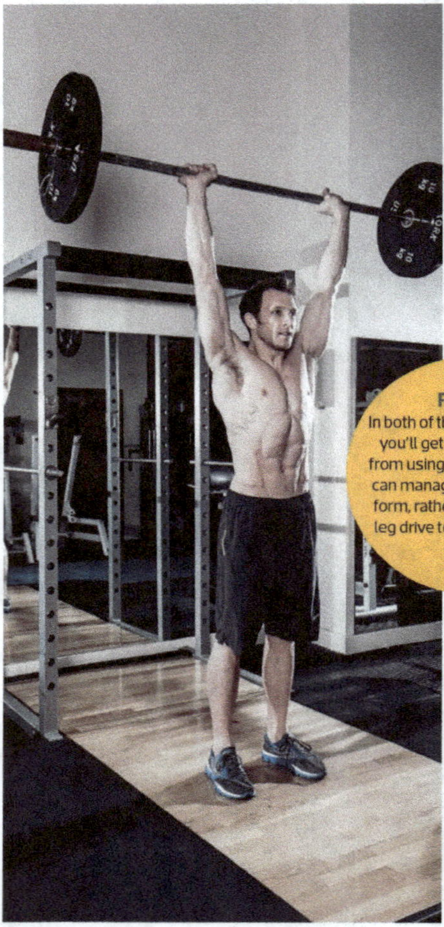

Hold the bar with your thumbs wrapped on the same side as your fingers, touching your shoulders. Brace your glutes and core and press the bar overhead, putting your head through the 'window' of your arms at the top. Lower under control.

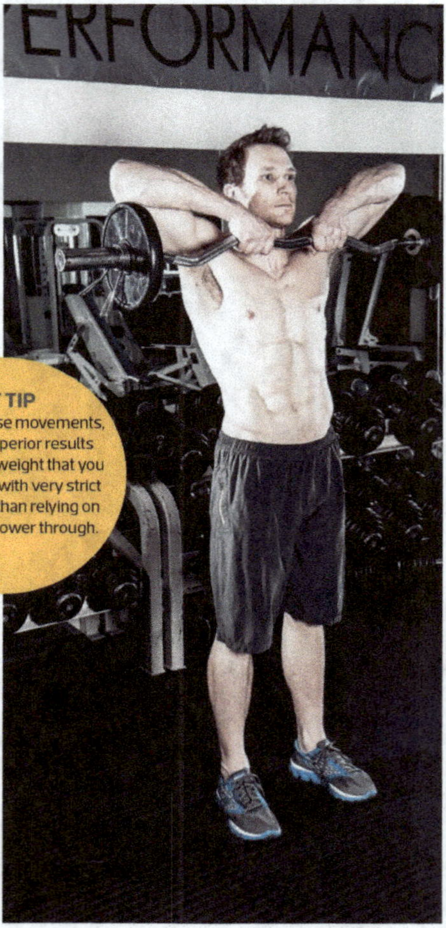

Hold an EZ-bar with your hands fairly close, palms facing you. Pull the bar up, bringing your elbows out to the sides, until it's under your chin. Pause, then lower. Don't use momentum – it's bad for your shoulders.

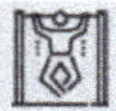

WORKOUT 4

  ## DB ARNOLD PRESS

SETS 3 REPS 8 TEMPO 1010 REST 60sec

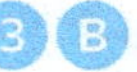 ## DB LATERAL RAISE

SETS 3 REPS 8 TEMPO 1010 REST 60sec

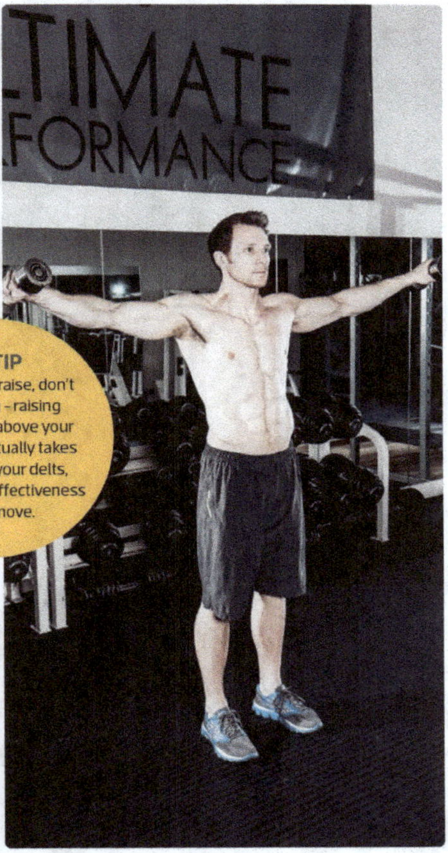

FIT TIP
In the lateral raise, don't go too high – raising the weights above your shoulders actually takes tension off your delts, reducing the effectiveness of the move.

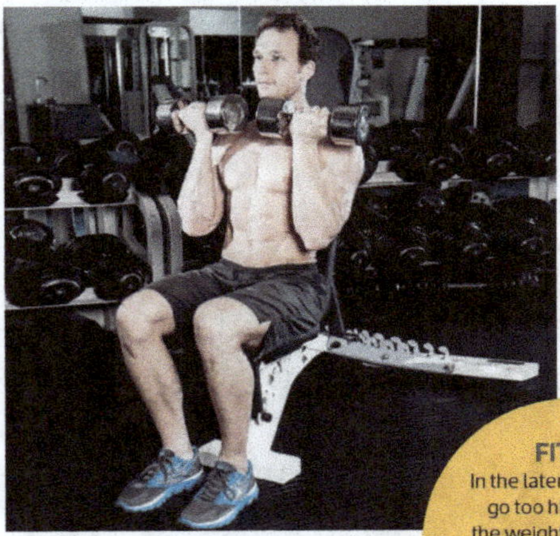

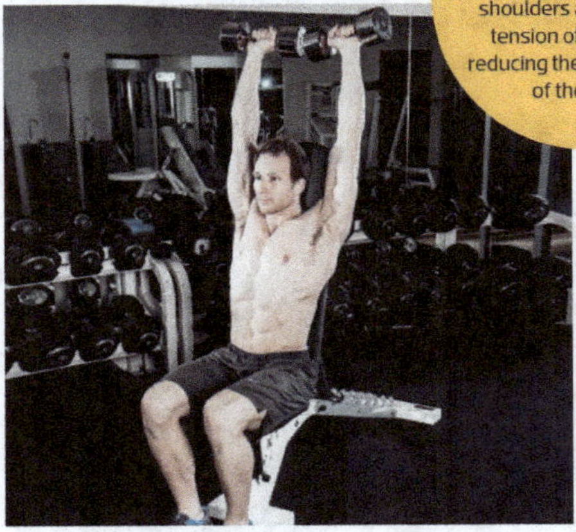

Sit on a bench holding dumbbells in the start position of a curl. Curl them upwards, then turn your palms away and press them overhead. Then reverse the whole movement to complete the rep.

Hold a light dumbbell in each hand. Raise them out to the sides, keeping a slight bend in your elbows. To keep the tension on the right muscles, keep your pinkies higher than your thumbs and don't go above shoulder height.

  BB SHRUG

SETS 3 REPS 8 TEMPO 1010 REST 60sec

Hold a heavy barbell with an overhand grip and 'shrug' your shoulders directly upwards – not in a circle. Pause, and then lower. If your grip becomes a limiting factor, use chalk or straps.

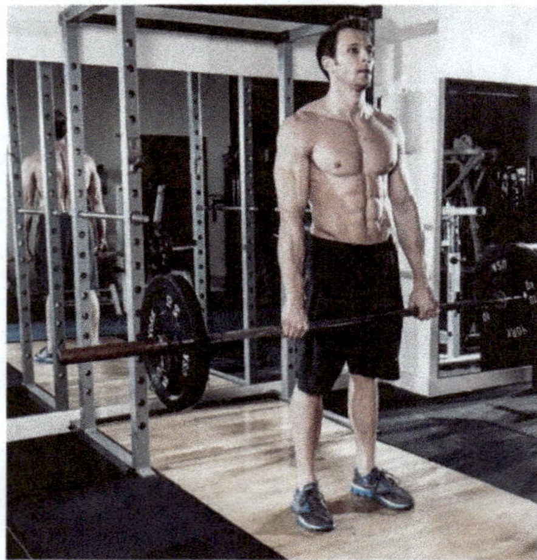 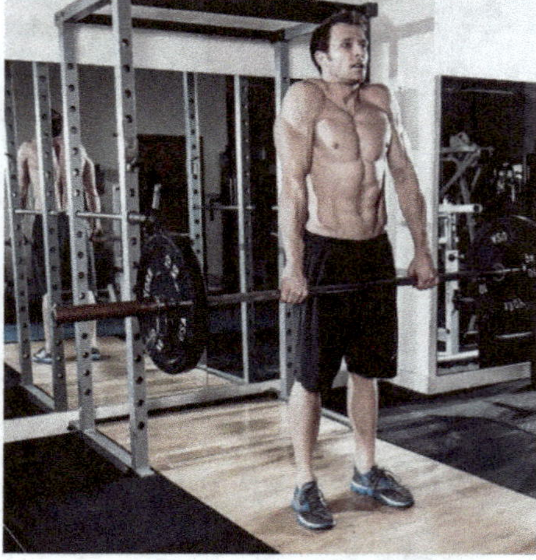

 PLANK

SETS 3 TIME 60sec REST 60sec

Get into a plank position with your forearms on the floor and hands clasped in front of you, then brace your abs and glutes to keep your body in a straight line. Hold that position.

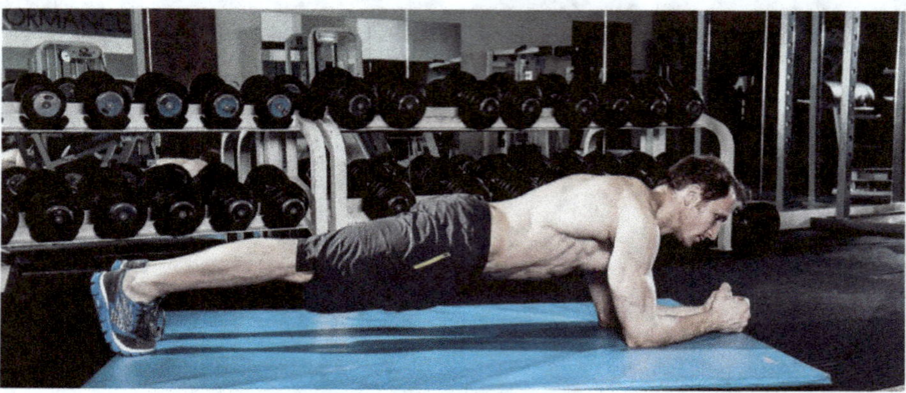

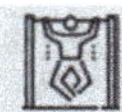

WEEK 2

Continue the body part split plan but up the reps to continue making gains

WORKOUT 1 **CHEST AND TRICEPS**

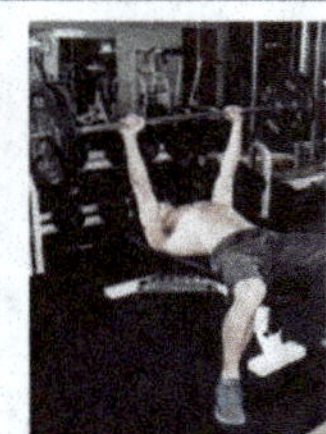

EXERCISE	SETS	REPS	TEMPO	REST
1 Bench press	5	12	1010	90SEC
2 Triceps dip	5	12	1010	90SEC
3A Incline dumbbell bench press	3	10	1010	60SEC
3B Incline dumbbell flye	3	10	1010	60SEC
4A Lying EZ-bar close-grip bench press	3	10	1010	60SEC
4B Lying EZ-bar triceps extension	3	10	1010	60SEC

WORKOUT 2 **BACK AND BICEPS**

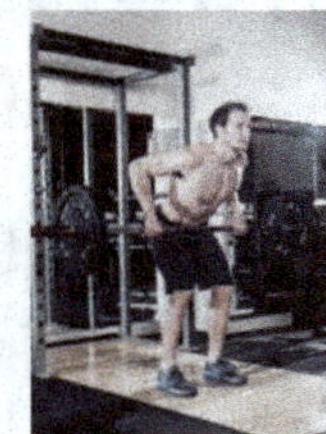

EXERCISE	SETS	REPS	TEMPO	REST
1 Bent-over row	5	12	1010	90SEC
2 Chin-up	5	12	1010	90SEC
3A Dumbbell one-arm bent-over row	3	10 EACH SIDE	1010	60SEC
3B Dumbbell one-arm bent-over flye	3	10 EACH SIDE	1010	60SEC
4A EZ-bar biceps curl	3	10	1010	60SEC
4B EZ-bar reverse curl	3	10	1010	60SEC

WORKOUT 3 **LEGS**

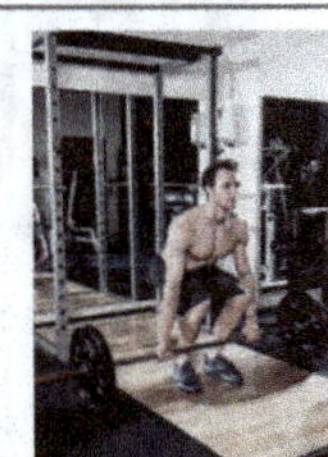

EXERCISE	SETS	REPS	TEMPO	REST
1 Deadlift	5	12	1010	90SEC
2 Squat	5	12	1010	90SEC
3A Dumbbell lunge	3	10 EACH SIDE	1010	60SEC
3B Dumbbell Romanian deadlift	3	10	1010	60SEC
4A Good morning	3	10	1010	60SEC
4B Glute bridge	3	10	1010	60SEC

WORKOUT 4 **SHOULDERS AND CORE**

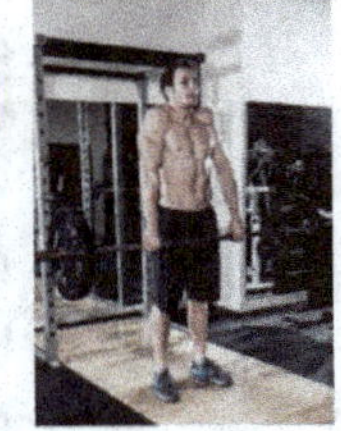

EXERCISE	SETS	REPS/TIME	TEMPO	REST
1 Overhead press	5	12	1010	90SEC
2 EZ-bar upright row	5	12	1010	90SEC
3A Dumbbell Arnold press	3	10	1010	60SEC
3B Dumbbell lateral raise	3	10	1010	60SEC
4A Barbell shrug	3	10	1010	60SEC
4B Plank	3	60SEC	1010	60SEC

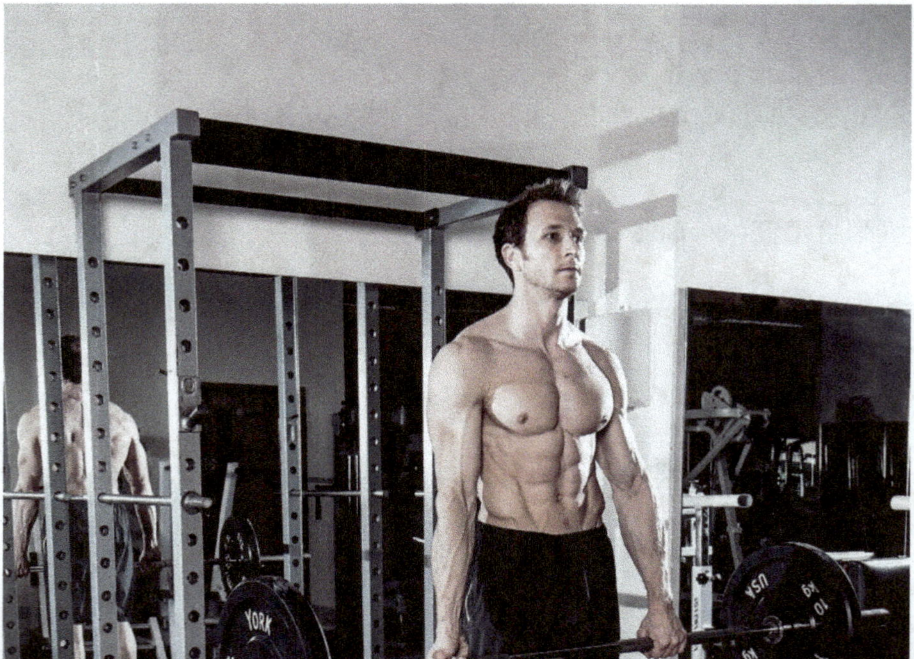

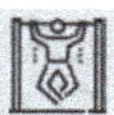

WEEK 3 WORKOUT 1

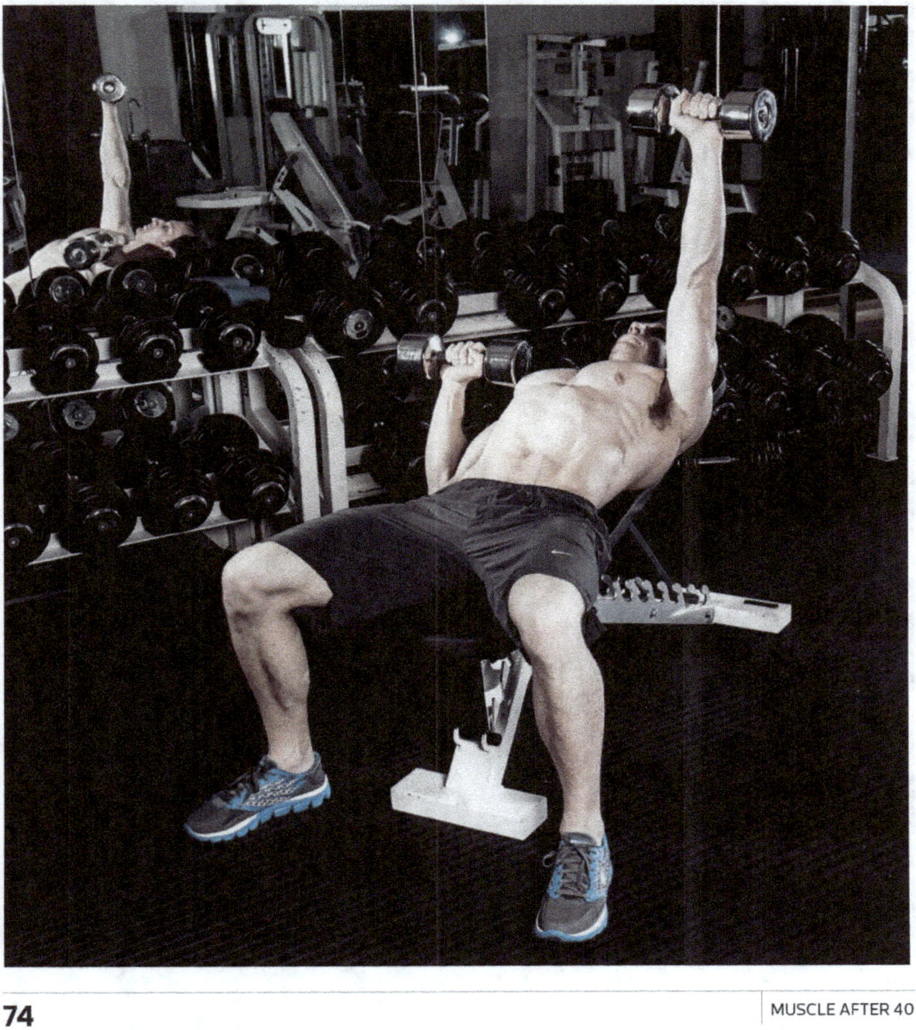

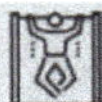

 INCLINE BENCH PRESS

SETS 5 REPS 10 TEMPO 1010 REST 90sec

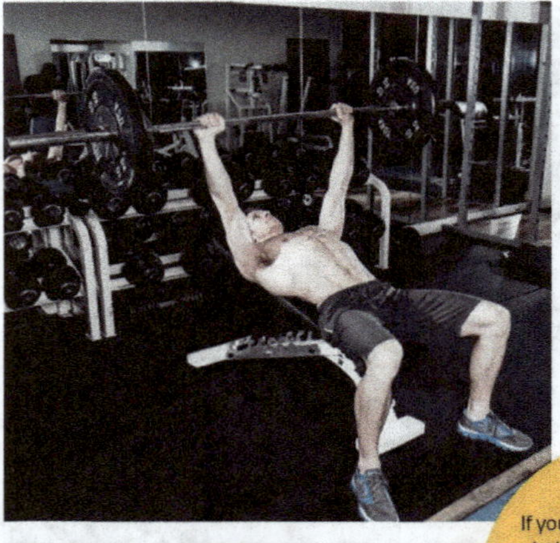

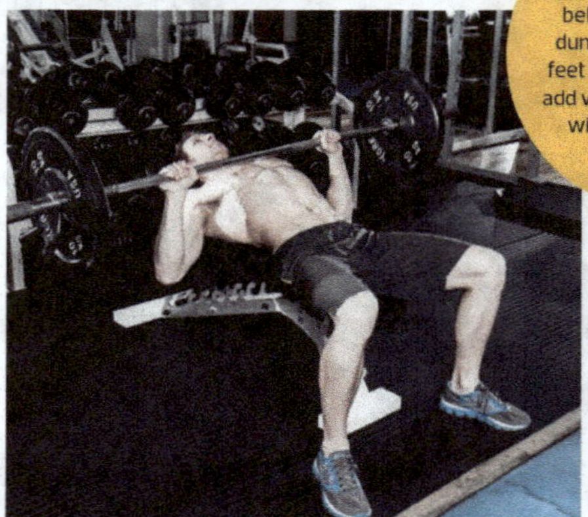

Lie on an incline bench with your feet on the floor.
Hold the bar with an overhand grip with your
hands shoulder-width apart. Slowly lower the bar
to your chest, then drive it strongly upwards.

 WEIGHTED TRICEPS DIP

SETS 5 REPS 10 TEMPO 1010 REST 90sec

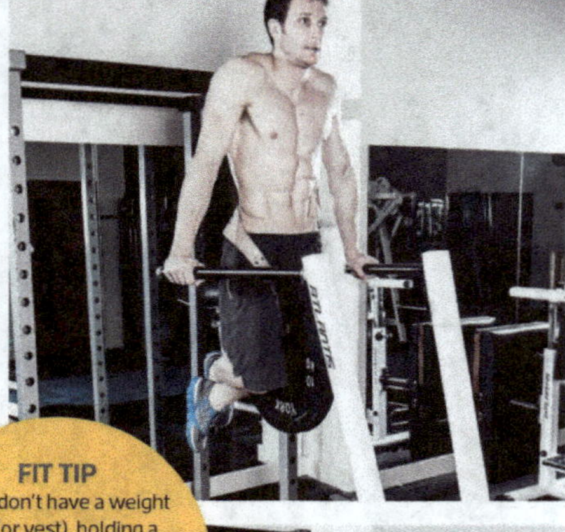

FIT TIP

If you don't have a weight
belt (or vest), holding a
dumbbell between your
feet is an excellent way to
add weight, if slightly tricky
with heavier weights.

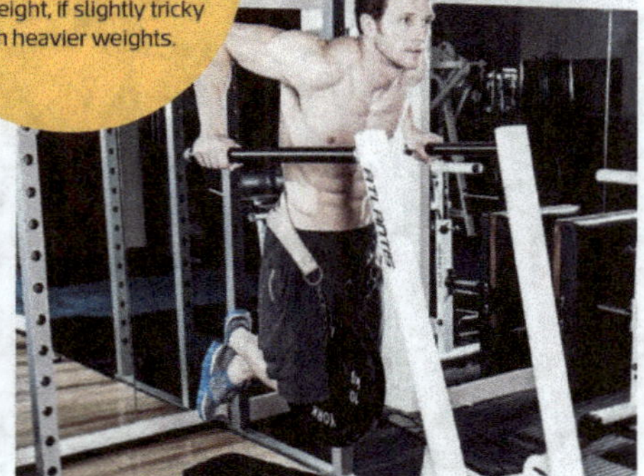

With a weight belt around your waist, grip a set of
dip bars with your hands roughly shoulder-width
apart, arms straight. Lower yourself until your
upper arms are parallel to the floor, keeping your
chest upright to hit your triceps. Press back up.

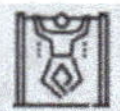

3 A ALTERNATING INCLINE BENCH

SETS 3 **REPS** 8 each side **TEMPO** 1010 **REST** 60sec

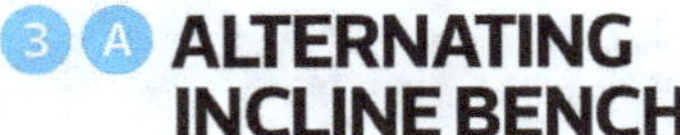

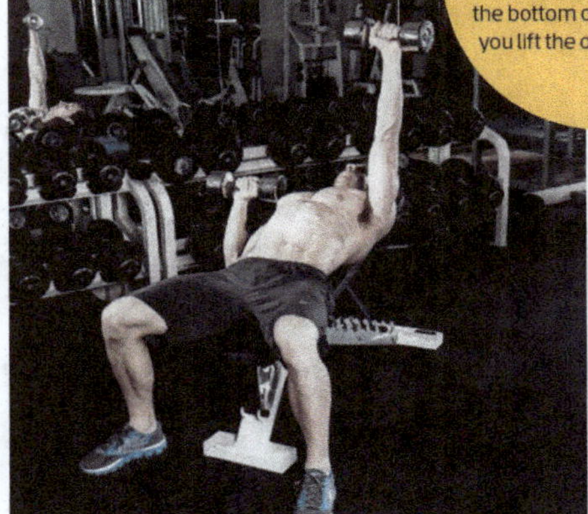

3 B LYING DB FLYE

SETS 3 **REPS** 8 **TEMPO** 1010 **REST** 60sec

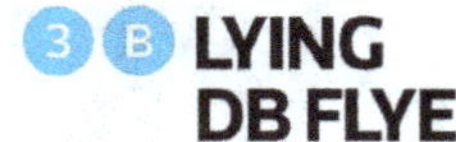

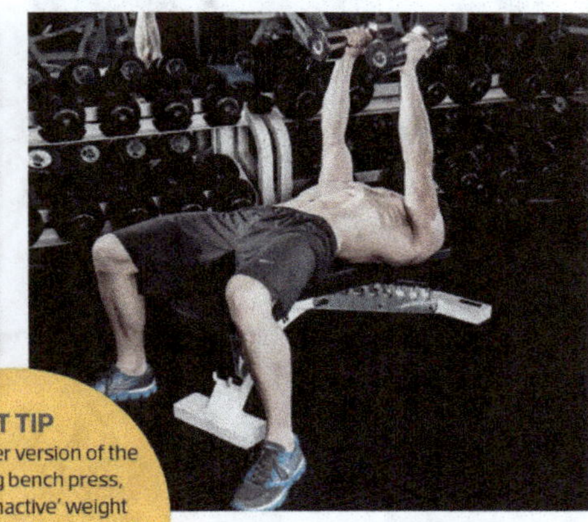

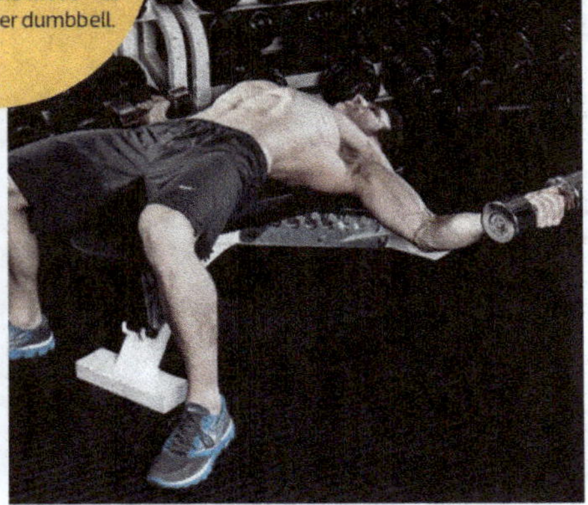

FIT TIP
For a tougher version of the alternating bench press, keep the 'inactive' weight overhead – rather than at the bottom of the move – as you lift the other dumbbell.

Lying on a bench set at an incline, press one dumbbell overhead, lower it and then repeat the move on the other side. This recruits more of the stabilising muscles of your torso in order to keep you steady.

Lie on a bench with the dumbbells above you, palms facing in. Bring your arms apart, keeping your elbows slightly bent, until you feel the stretch in your chest, then bring them back together.

4 A EZ-BAR PULL-OVER

SETS 3 REPS 8 TEMPO 1010 REST 60sec

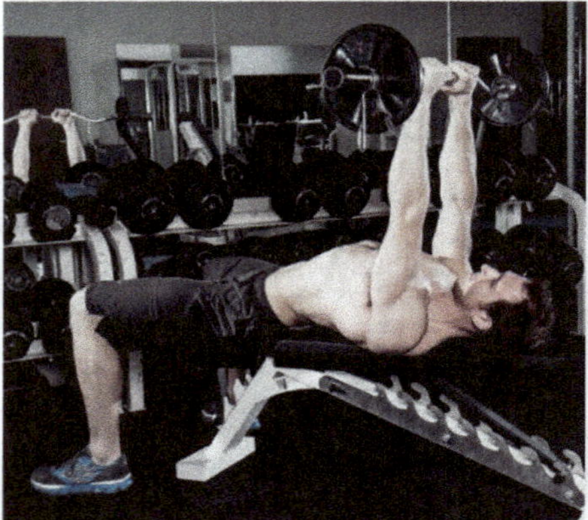

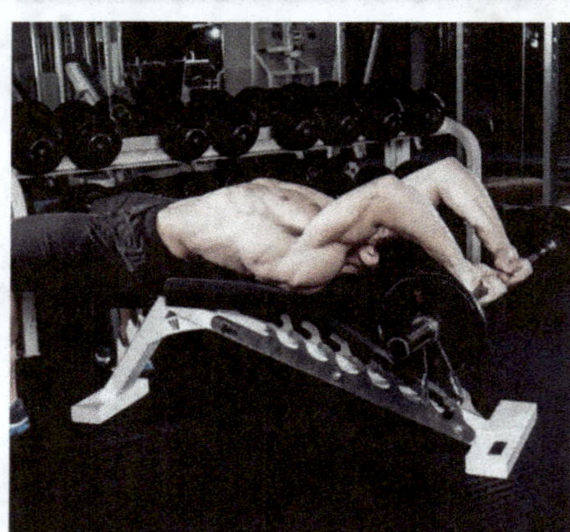

Lie on a bench with an EZ-bar held overhead. Keeping a slight bend in your arms, lower the weight behind your head until you feel the stretch in your triceps, pause and then pull it back over your head.

4 B CLOSE-GRIP BENCH PRESS

SETS 3 REPS 8 TEMPO 1010 REST 60sec

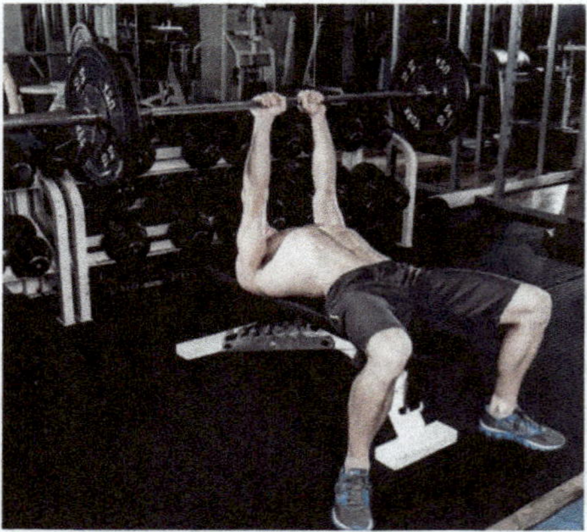

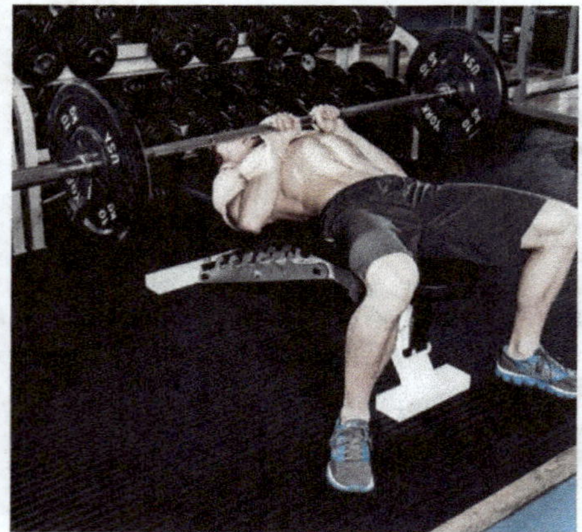

Lie on a bench and grip a barbell with your hands just narrower than shoulder-width apart. Lower the barbell to your chest, keeping your elbows close to your sides. Pause, and then press back up.

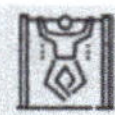

WORKOUT 2

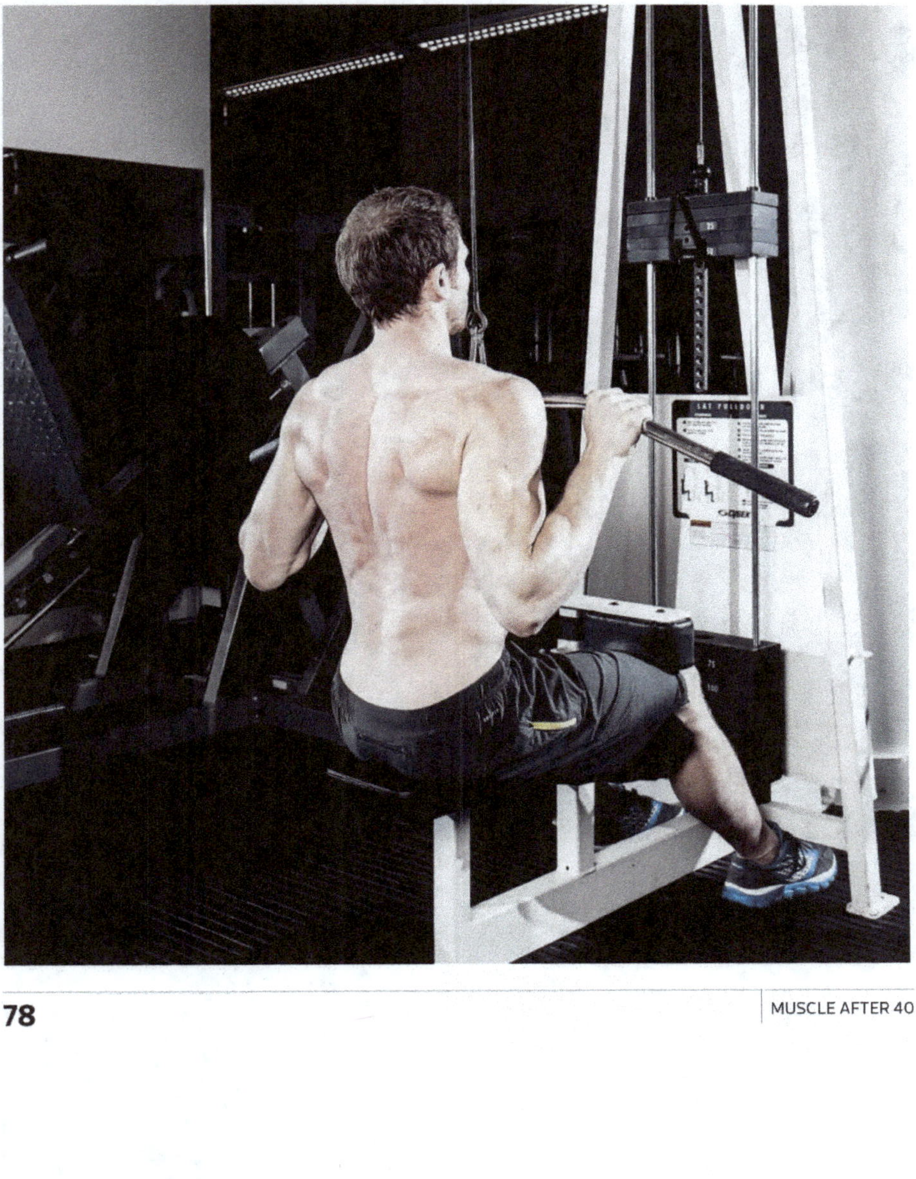

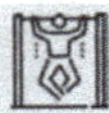

① BENT-OVER ROW

SETS 5 **REPS** 10 **TEMPO** 1010 **REST** 90sec

② WEIGHTED CHIN-UP

SETS 5 **REPS** 6–10 **TEMPO** 1010 **REST** 90sec

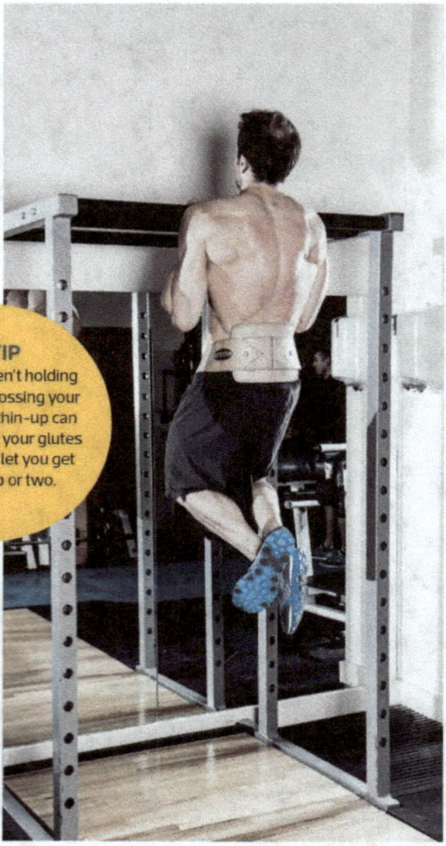

FIT TIP
Even if you aren't holding a dumbbell, crossing your feet during a chin-up can help you brace your glutes and core, and let you get another rep or two.

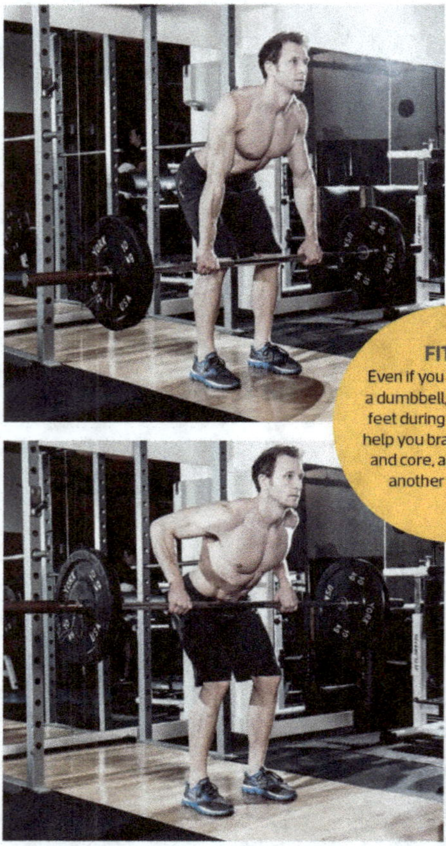

Bend your knees slightly and lean forwards with your hands just wider than shoulder-width apart on the bar. Pull the bar up to your lower sternum, focusing on pulling your elbows behind you, then lower under control.

Wearing a weight belt or vest or holding a dumbbell between your feet, hang from a bar with palms facing you. Pull up until your chin's over the bar. Pause, then lower – don't drop, or you'll risk hurting your elbows at the bottom.

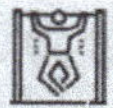

WORKOUT 2

3 A WIDE-GRIP PULL-DOWN

SETS 3 **REPS** 8 **TEMPO** 1010 **REST** 60sec

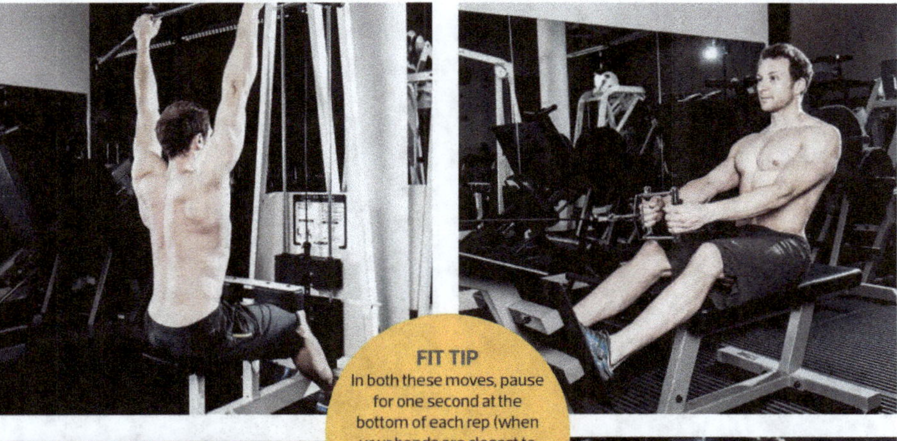

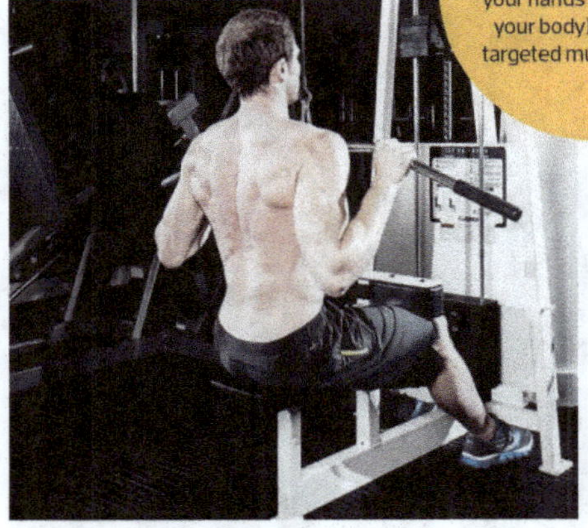

3 B SEATED ROW

SETS 3 **REPS** 8 **TEMPO** 1010 **REST** 60sec

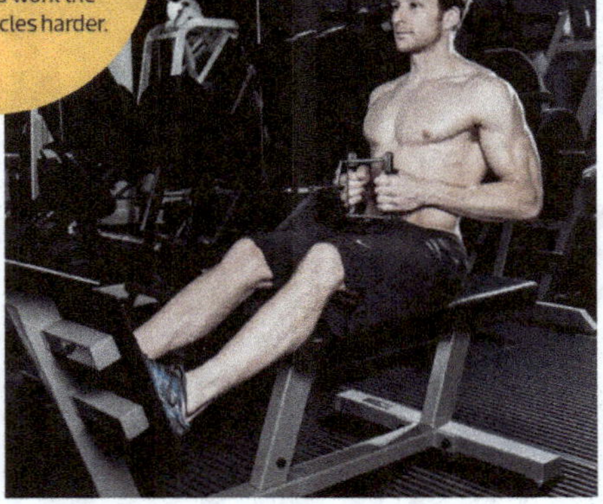

FIT TIP
In both these moves, pause for one second at the bottom of each rep (when your hands are closest to your body) to work the targeted muscles harder.

Sit on the pull-down machine and take a wide grip on the bar, hands almost double shoulder-width apart. Pull the bar down to your chest, aiming to bring your elbows behind you. Focus on keeping your shoulder blades engaged.

Sit on the machine with a double-D handle attached, knees slightly bent. Pull the handle in to your sternum, bringing your elbows behind you and your shoulder blades together. Pause, then return to the start position.

4 A EZ-BAR BICEPS CURL

SETS 3 **REPS** 8 **TEMPO** 1010 **REST** 60sec

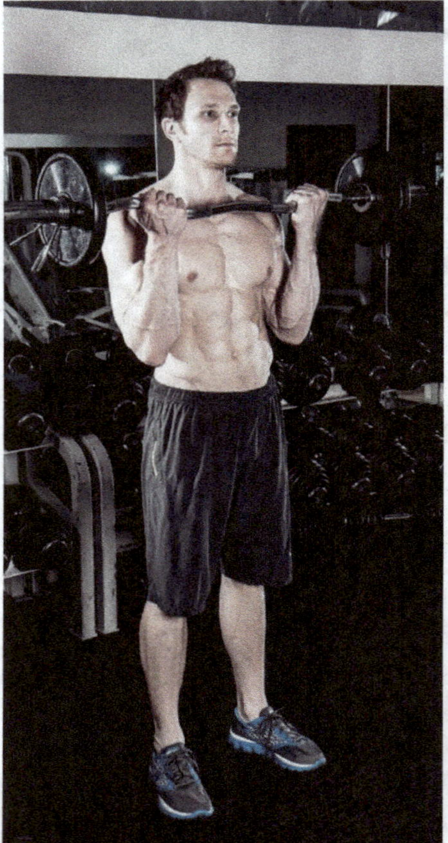

Using an EZ-bar reduces stress on your elbows. Stand straight and curl the bar upwards. Squeeze your biceps at the top of the movement and your triceps at the bottom.

4 B DB HAMMER CURL

SETS 3 **REPS** 8 **TEMPO** 1010 **REST** 60sec

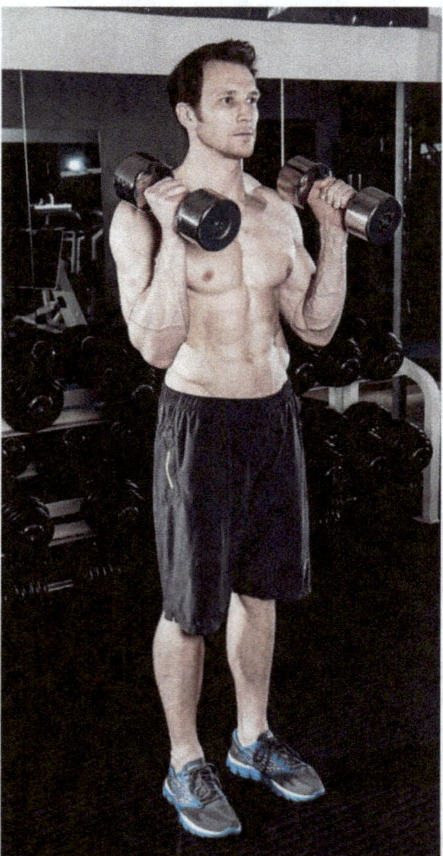

Start by holding dumbbells, palms facing your thighs. Curl both weights up, squeezing your biceps at the top of the move. Don't alternate arms – this takes too much tension off the muscle while one arm rests.

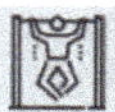

WORKOUT 3

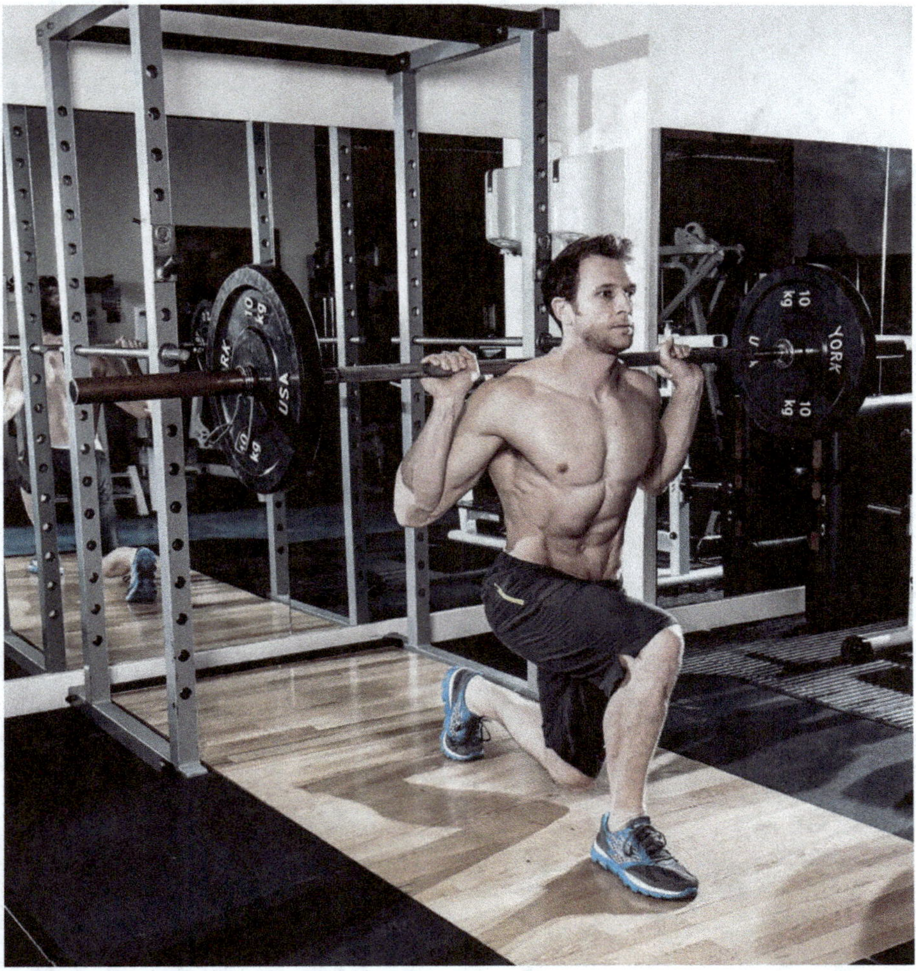

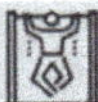

① SUMO SQUAT

SETS 5 **REPS** 10 **TEMPO** 1010 **REST** 90sec

② FRONT SQUAT

SETS 5 **REPS** 10 **TEMPO** 1010 **REST** 90sec

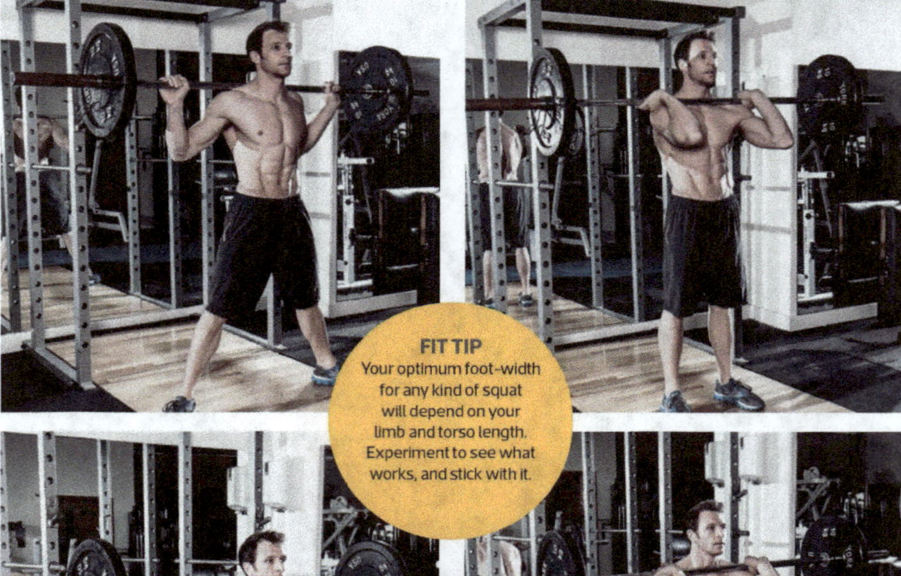

FIT TIP
Your optimum foot-width for any kind of squat will depend on your limb and torso length. Experiment to see what works, and stick with it.

Start with a barbell across your back and your feet wider than in a traditional squat, toes pointed out to the sides. Lower into a squat, pause when your thighs are parallel to the ground, then stand up straight.

Grip the barbell with hands slightly wider than shoulder-width apart and elbows pointing forwards. Unrack the bar, take a deep breath, brace your core and lower under control into a full squat. Drive back up through your midfoot to stand.

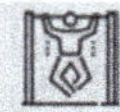

WORKOUT 3

  ## BB SQUAT

SETS 3 REPS 8 TEMPO 1010 REST 60sec

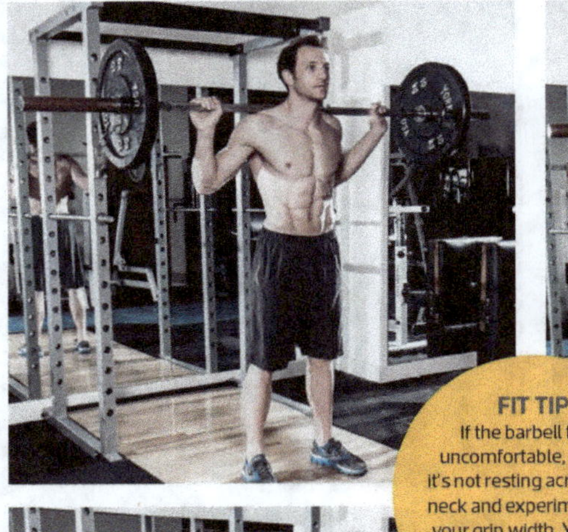

Stand with your feet just wider than shoulder-width apart, holding the bar on your upper traps. Sit down and back, keeping your chest up and your core engaged. When you've gone as low as possible, drive through your heels to stand.

3 B BB LUNGE

SETS 3 REPS 8 each side TEMPO 1010 REST 60sec

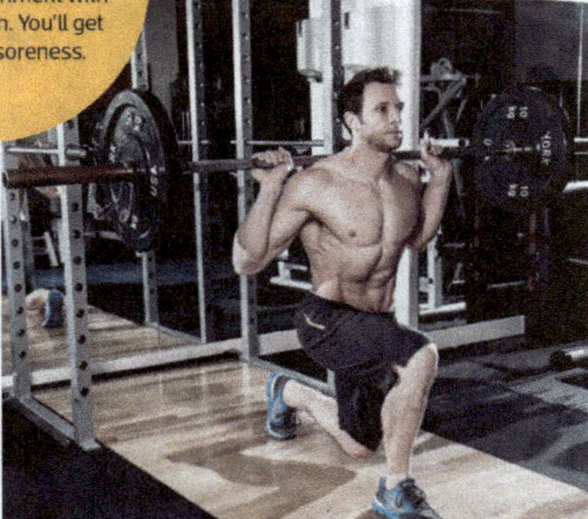

Stand holding the barbell across your traps and take a big lunge forward, allowing your trailing knee to brush the floor. Push off your front foot to return to the start, and repeat on the other side.

FIT TIP
If the barbell feels uncomfortable, ensure it's not resting across your neck and experiment with your grip width. You'll get used to the soreness.

  ROMANIAN DEADLIFT GLUTE BRIDGE

SETS 3 REPS 8 TEMPO 1010 REST 60sec **SETS 3 REPS 8 TEMPO 1010 REST 60sec**

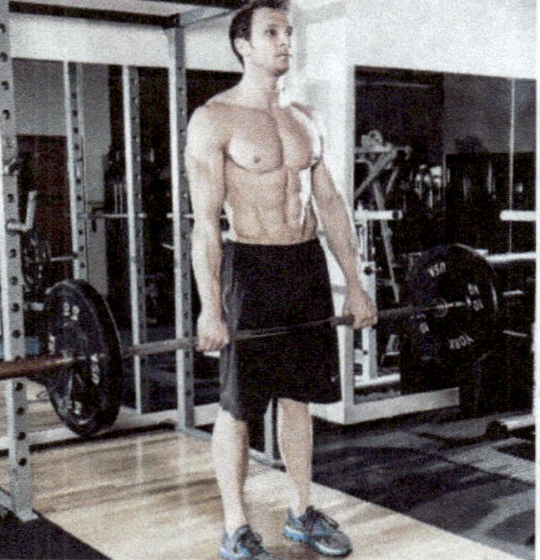

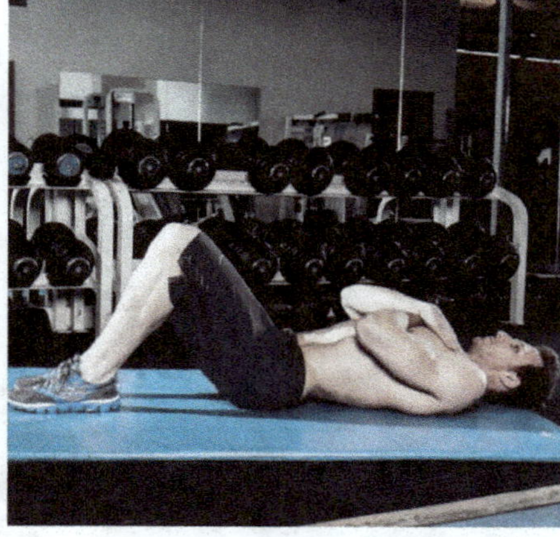

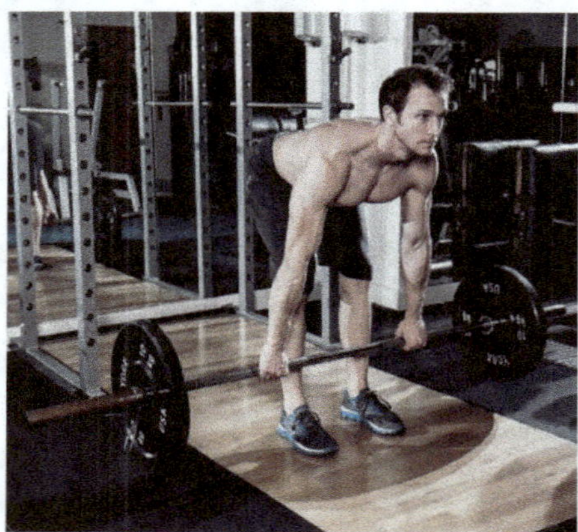

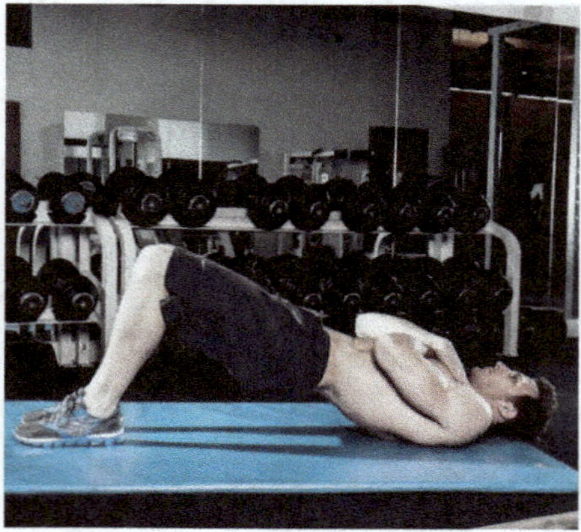

Grab the bar with an overhand grip. Bend your knees slightly, then keep your chest up, shoulders back and maintain a neutral arch in your lower back as you push your hips back. Go as far as you can while keeping the bar close to your body.

Lie on the floor with your feet close to your glutes. Drive through your heels to raise your hips, tense your glutes at the top of the move, then lower under control. If it's too easy, add a weight plate or barbell.

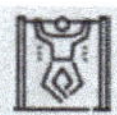

WORKOUT 4

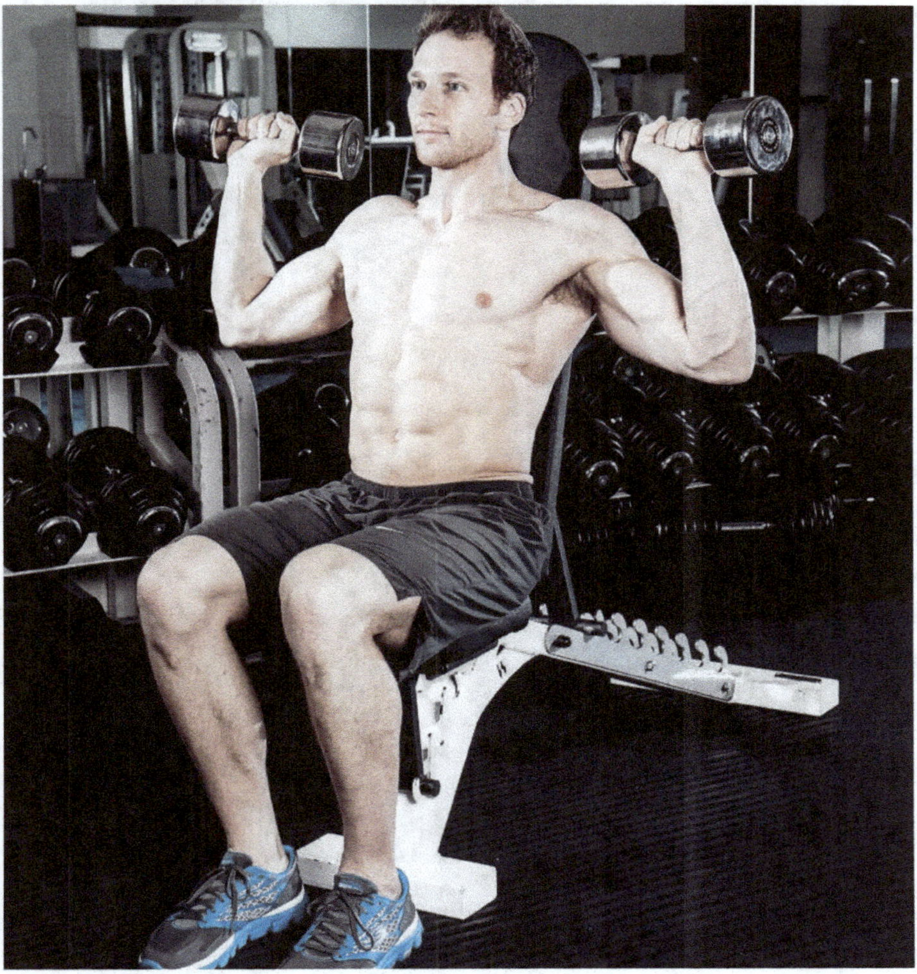

① PUSH PRESS

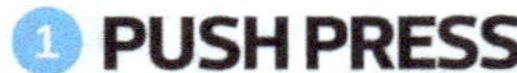

SETS 5 **REPS** 10 **TEMPO** 1010 **REST** 90sec

② BB SHRUG

SETS 5 **REPS** 10 **TEMPO** 1010 **REST** 90sec

FIT TIP
If you haven't got any straps, try a trap bar – it'll take some of the emphasis off your grip and allow you to handle more weight than a straight-bar shrug.

Hold the bar at shoulder level. Do a quarter-squat to gather momentum, then drive explosively through your heels to help you press the bar overhead. Pause at the top, and lower under control.

Hold a heavy barbell with an overhand grip and 'shrug' your shoulders directly upwards - not in a circle. Pause, and then lower. If your grip becomes a limiting factor, use chalk or straps.

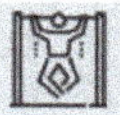

WORKOUT 4

3 A SEATED DB PRESS

SETS 3 **REPS** 8 **TEMPO** 1010 **REST** 60sec

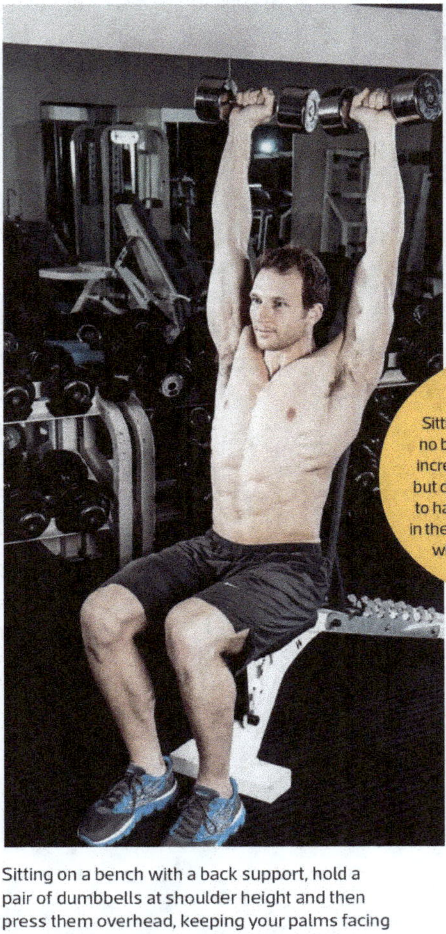

Sitting on a bench with a back support, hold a pair of dumbbells at shoulder height and then press them overhead, keeping your palms facing forward. Don't lock out completely at the top – it'll keep the tension on your tris and delts.

3 B DB LATERAL RAISE

SETS 3 **REPS** 8 **TEMPO** 1010 **REST** 60sec

FIT TIP
Sitting on a bench with no backrest will slightly increase core activation, but decrease your abilitiy to handle heavy weights in the shoulder press. Pick what works for you.

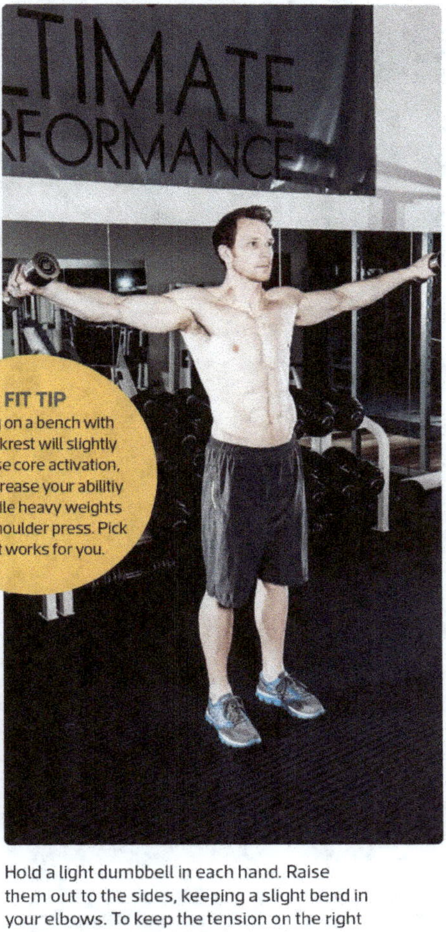

Hold a light dumbbell in each hand. Raise them out to the sides, keeping a slight bend in your elbows. To keep the tension on the right muscles, keep your pinkies higher than your thumbs and don't go above shoulder height.

4 A EZ-BAR UPRIGHT ROW 4 B PLANK

SETS 3 **REPS** 8 **TEMPO** 1010 **REST** 60sec

SETS 3 **TIME** 60sec **REST** 60sec

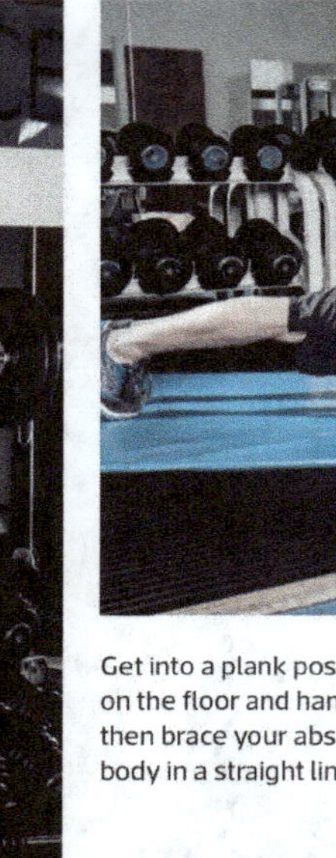

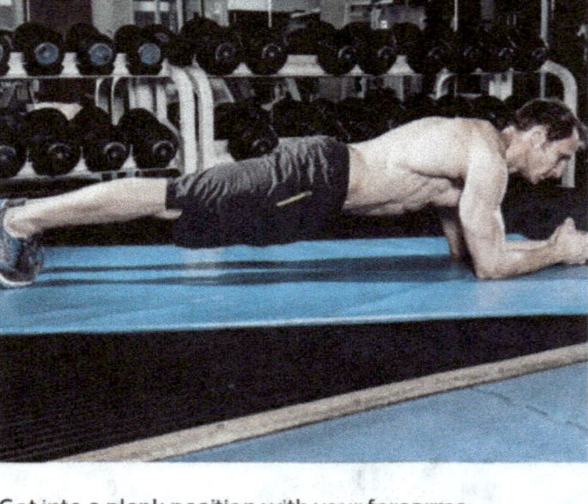

Get into a plank position with your forearms on the floor and hands clasped in front of you, then brace your abs and glutes to keep your body in a straight line. Hold that position.

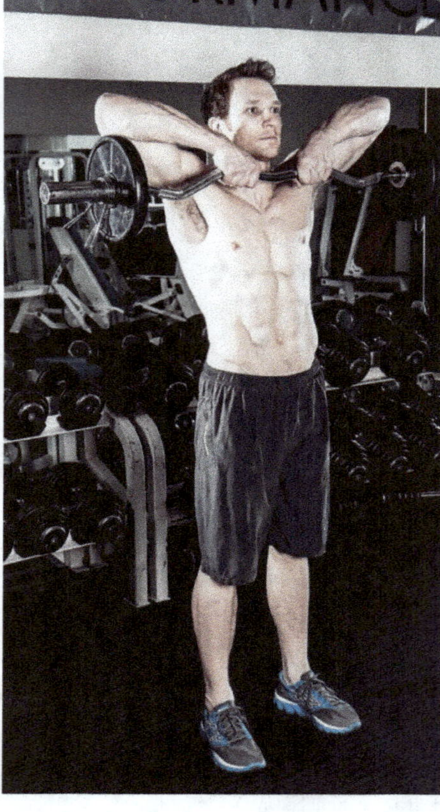

Hold an EZ-bar with your hands fairly close, palms facing you. Pull the bar up, bringing your elbows out to the sides, until it's under your chin. Pause, then lower. Don't use momentum – it's bad for your shoulders.

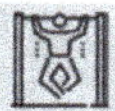

WEEK 4

The final week of your strength phase ups the volume. Make sure you keep those rests strict

WORKOUT 1 **CHEST AND TRICEPS**

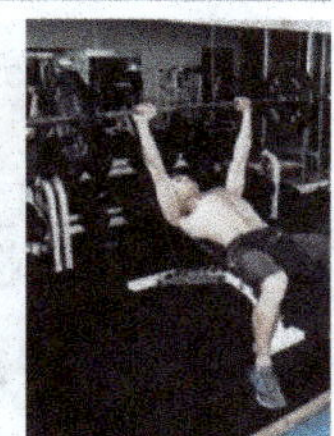

EXERCISE	SETS	REPS	TEMPO	REST
1 Incline bench press	5	12	1010	90SEC
2 Weighted triceps dip	5	12	1010	90SEC
3A Alternating incline bench press	3	10 EACH SIDE	1010	60SEC
3B Lying dumbbell flye	3	10	1010	60SEC
4A EZ-bar pull-over	3	10	1010	60SEC
4B Close-grip bench press	3	10	1010	60SEC

WORKOUT 2 **BACK AND BICEPS**

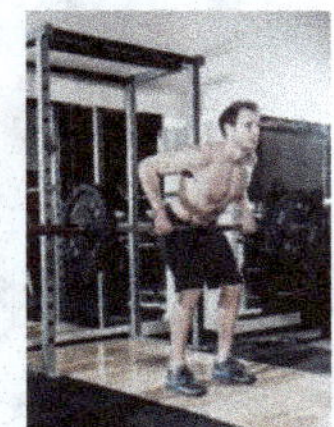

EXERCISE	SETS	REPS	TEMPO	REST
1 Bent-over row	5	12	1010	90SEC
2 Weighted chin-up	5	12	1010	90SEC
3A Wide-grip lat pull-down	3	10	1010	60SEC
3B Seated row	3	10	1010	60SEC
4A EZ-bar biceps curl	3	10	1010	60SEC
4B Dumbbell hammer curl	3	10	1010	60SEC

WORKOUT 3 **LEGS**

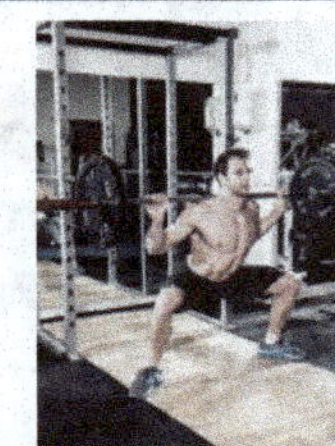

EXERCISE	SETS	REPS	TEMPO	REST
1 Sumo squat	5	12	1010	90SEC
2 Front squat	5	12	1010	90SEC
3A Squat	3	10	1010	60SEC
3B Barbell lunge	3	10 EACH SIDE	1010	60SEC
4A Romanian deadlift	3	10	1010	60SEC
4B Glute bridge	3	10	1010	60SEC

WORKOUT 4 **SHOULDERS AND CORE**

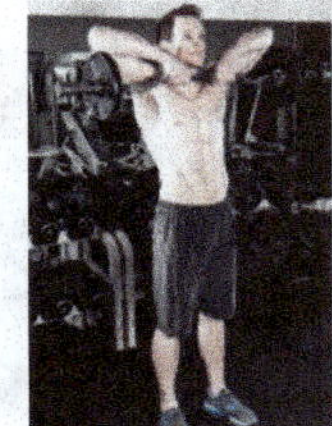

EXERCISE	SETS	REPS/TIME	TEMPO	REST
1 Push press	5	12	1010	90SEC
2 Barbell shrug	5	12	1010	90SEC
3A Seated dumbbell overhead press	3	10	1010	60SEC
3B Dumbbell lateral raise	3	10	1010	60SEC
4A EZ-bar upright row	3	10	1010	60SEC
4B Plank	3	60SEC	1010	60SEC

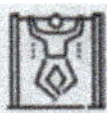

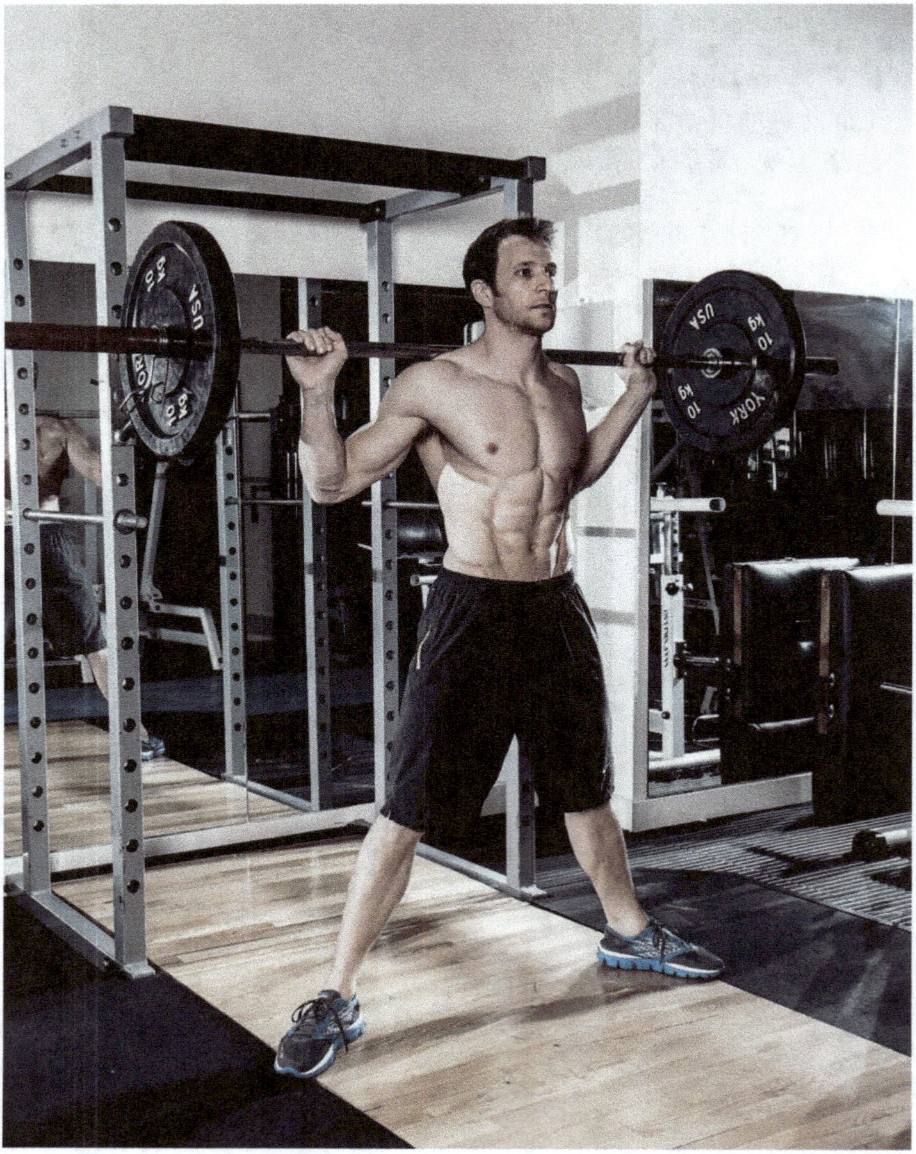

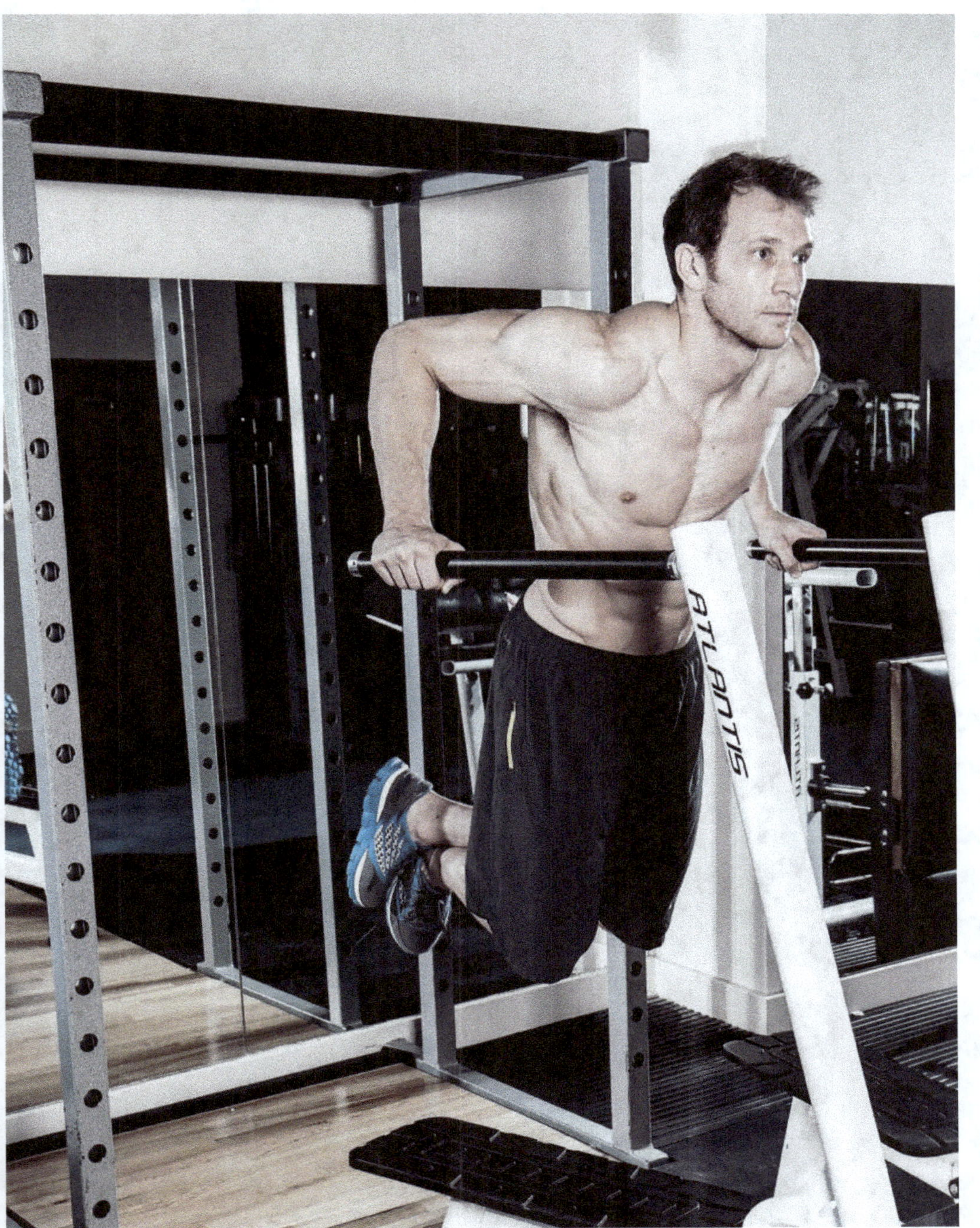

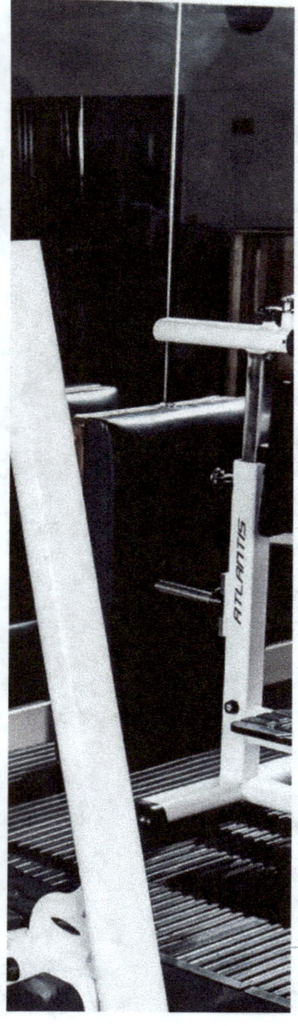

THE FINAL PUSH

In the last four weeks of your plan you'll push your muscles to the limit. Go hard, then go home

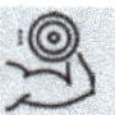

GAINS WITH BRAINS

In the final phase of your programme, the intensity ramps up and the rests go down. This time, every session includes three pairs of movements done as supersets, forcing you to work at a high pace throughout each workout (and helping you burn fat to ensure your hard-earned muscle stays on display). This time, though, you'll focus on antagonistic supersets, in which you work opposing muscle groups which allows you to pack in more work in less time.

Thanks to an effect called reciprocal innervation, it also means you'll be able to work harder. Research suggests that when you're working one muscle group, the 'antagonist' muscle (which performs the opposite function) rests, allowing it to work harder in its next set –triceps and biceps, for example. Again, where the exercises are marked A and B, you do one set of move A, rest as indicated, then one set of B, then rest, and continue till you complete all the reps. The rests are shorter now too.

This phase also introduces more cable movements. These are key because they keep tension on the muscle throughout the entire range of motion for each rep. And finally, there's more core training, giving you a more stable base to do your pressing and squatting from. This is where all the hard work you've put in pays dividends - keep working hard, but remember to enjoy it.

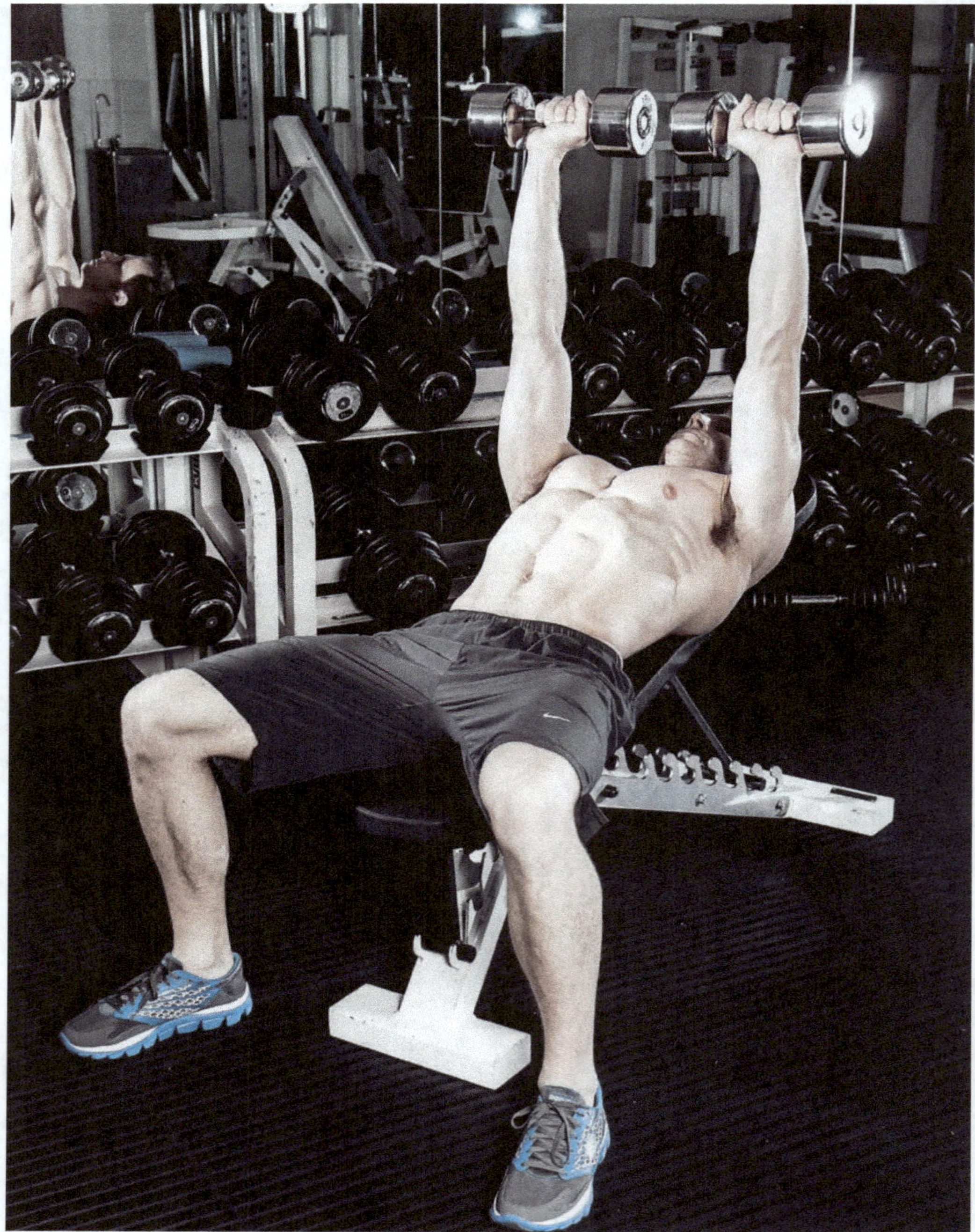

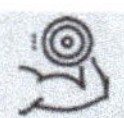

WEEK 1 WORKOUT 1

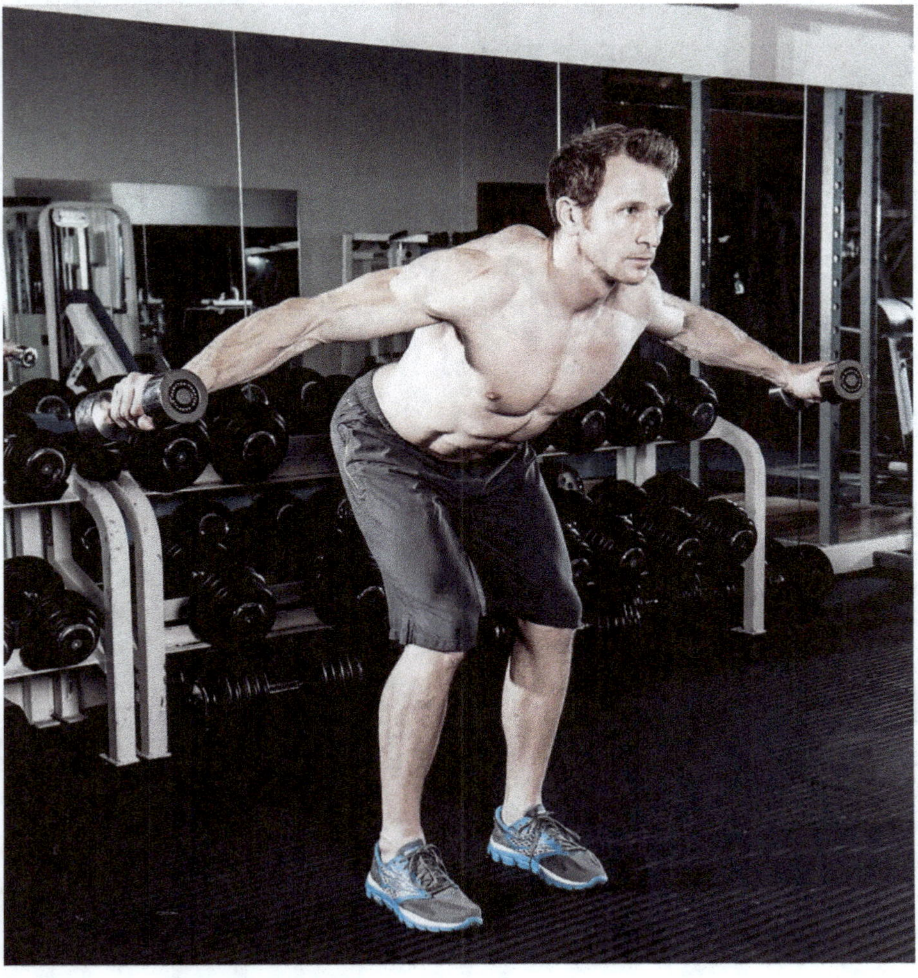

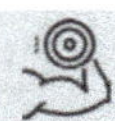

1 A INCLINE DB BENCH PRESS

SETS 5 REPS 8 TEMPO 2010 REST 10sec

1 B DB ONE-ARM BENT-OVER ROW

SETS 5 REPS 8 each side TEMPO 2110 REST 45sec

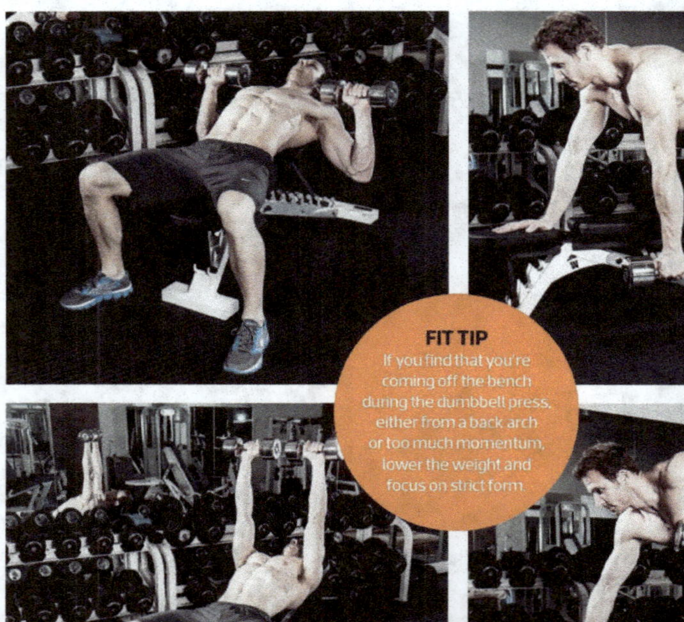

Lie on a bench set at a 30° angle holding a dumbbell in each hand. Keep your feet flat on the floor and your back against the bench. Press the weights straight up, without locking out at the top, then lower.

Place one knee on a bench, supporting your torso with a straight arm, holding a dumbbell in the other hand. With your foot flat and core braced, row the weight up, leading with your elbow, then lower. Do all the reps on one side, then switch.

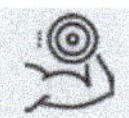

WORKOUT 1

2A CABLE CROSS-OVER

SETS 4 REPS 10 TEMPO 2010 REST 10sec

2B LAT PULL-DOWN

SETS 4 REPS 10 TEMPO 2010 REST 45sec

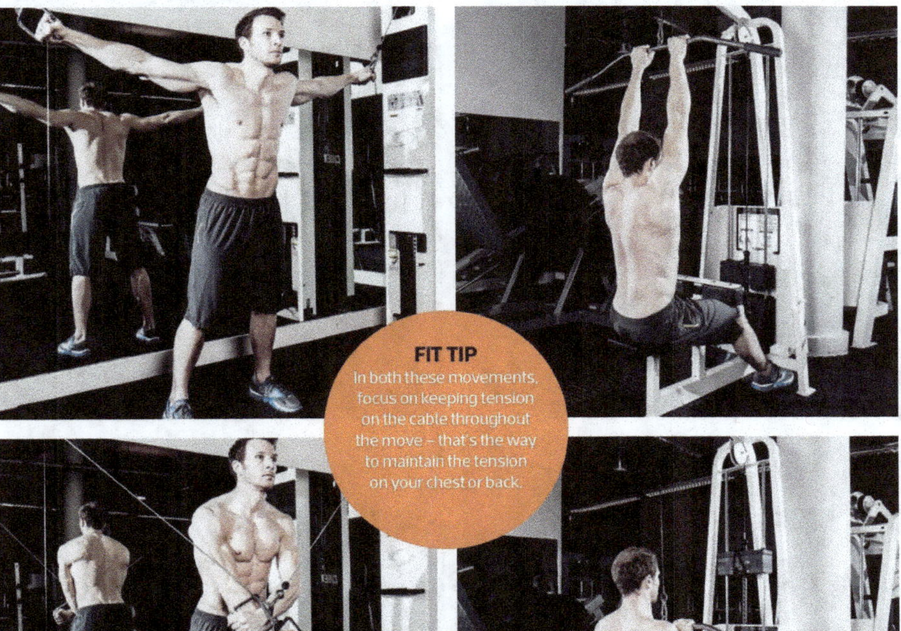

Stand with a split stance holding a D–handle attachment in each hand, with the cable set above shoulder height. Bring your hands down in an arc to meet in front of your chest, squeeze your chest muscles, then return to the start.

Sit on the pull–down machine and grip the bar with your arms vertical. Pull the bar down to your chest, aiming to bring your elbows down and behind you. Focus on keeping your shoulders engaged.

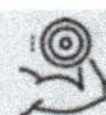

3 A CABLE FLYE

SETS 3 REPS 12 TEMPO 2111 REST 10sec

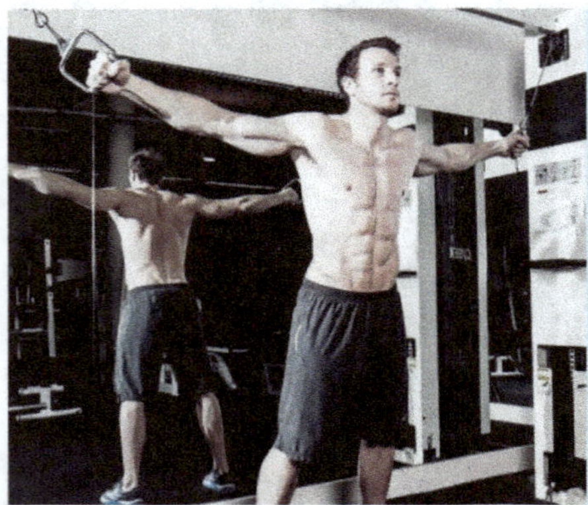

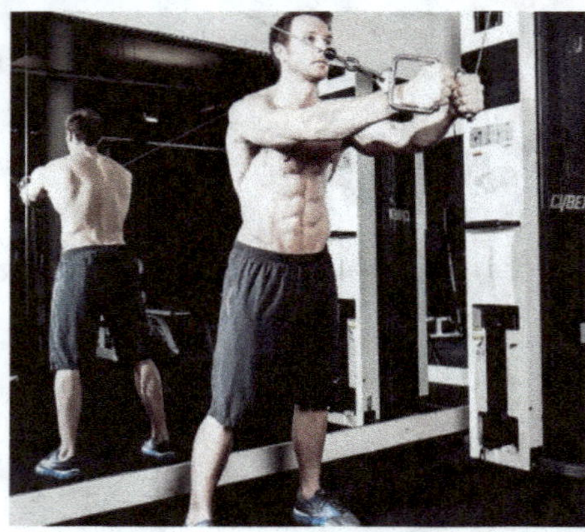

Hold the cable D-handles as you would in the cross-over, but this time keep them at shoulder height, bringing your hands together and squeezing your chest muscles at the end of the movement.

3 B BENT-OVER REVERSE FLYE

SETS 3 REPS 12 TEMPO 2111 REST 45sec

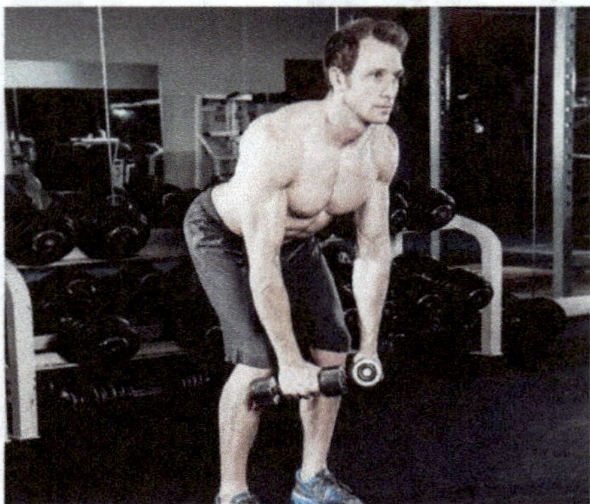

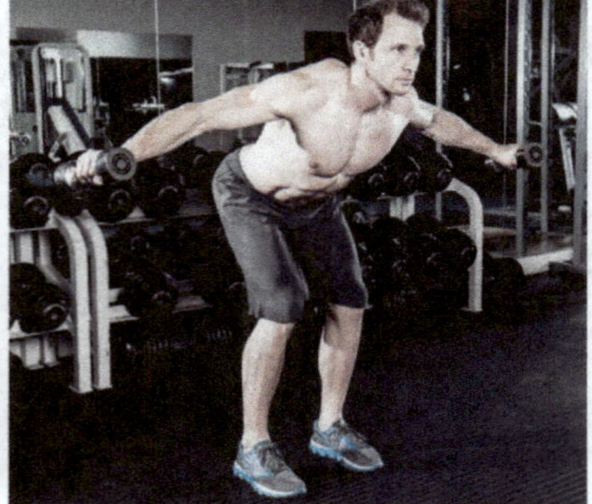

Holding a pair of dumbbells, bend forwards at the hips and, keeping a slight bend in your elbows, raise them to your sides as if spreading your wings, pulling your shoulder blades together.

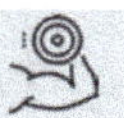

WORKOUT 2

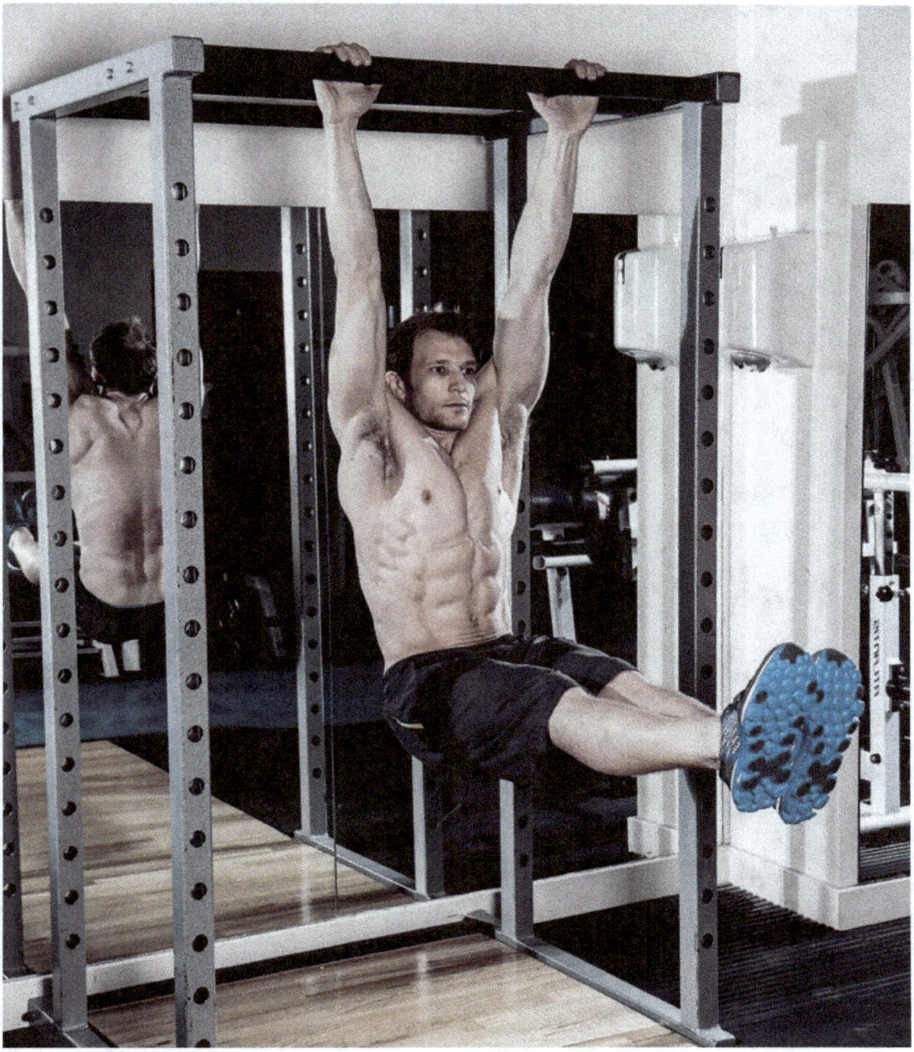

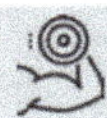

1 A BB LUNGE

SETS 5 REPS 8 each side TEMPO 2010 REST 10sec

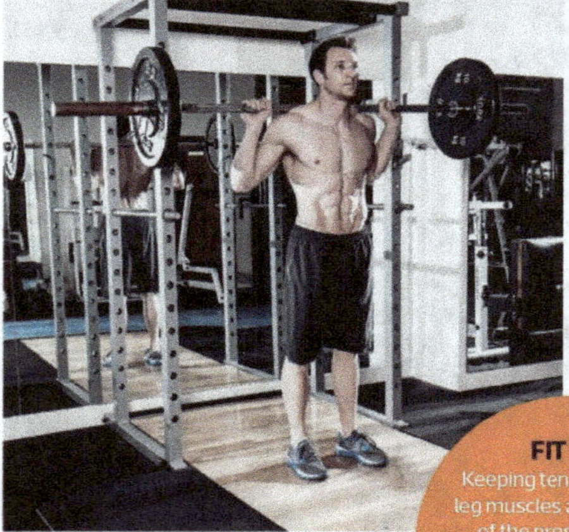

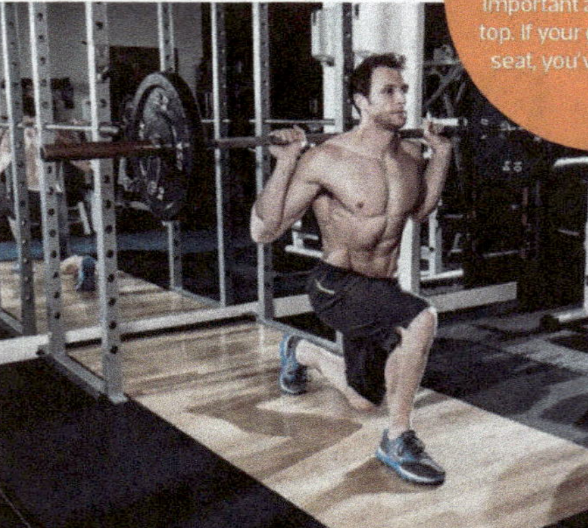

Stand holding the barbell across your traps and take a big lunge forward, allowing your trailing knee to brush the floor. Push off your front foot to return to the start, and repeat on the other side.

1 B LEG PRESS

SETS 5 REPS 8 TEMPO 2010 REST 45sec

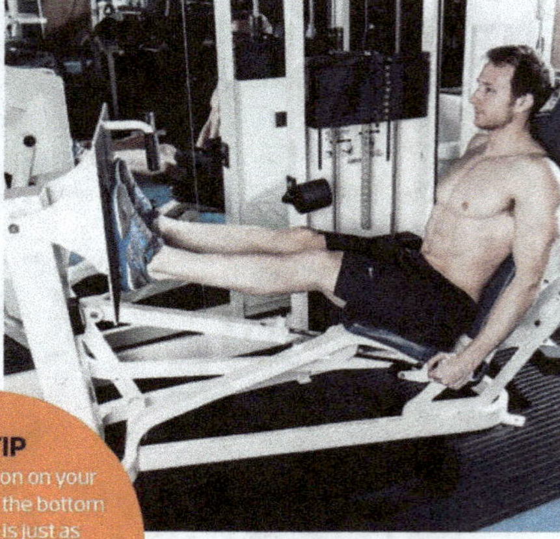

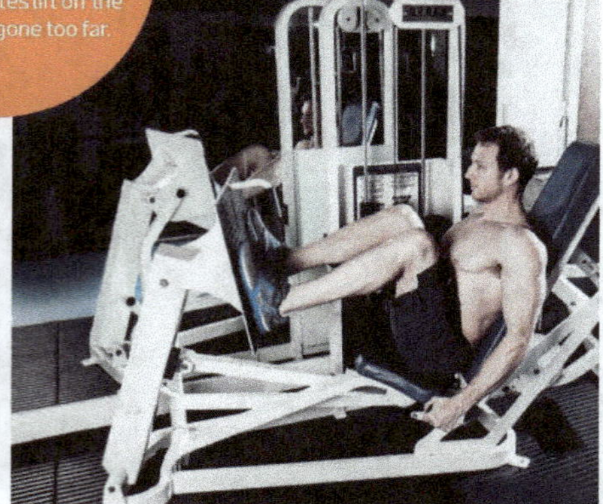

FIT TIP
Keeping tension on your leg muscles at the bottom of the press is just as important as doing it at the top. If your glutes lift off the seat, you've gone too far.

Sit on the machine, release the lock then slowly lower the platform until your legs are at 90°. Pause briefly at the bottom, then push through your heels to straighten your legs. Don't lock out fully at the top.

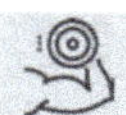

WORKOUT 2

  GOBLET SQUAT

SETS 4 **REPS** 10 **TEMPO** 2010 **REST** 10sec

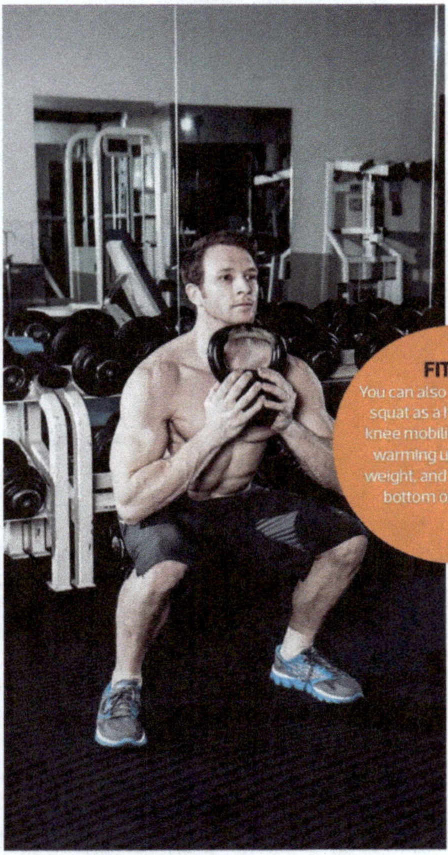

  DB STEP-UP

SETS 4 **REPS** 10 each side **TEMPO** 2010 **REST** 45sec

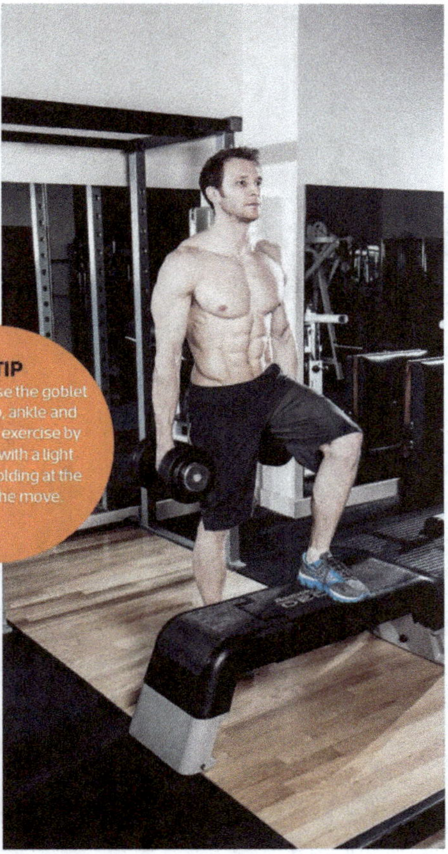

FIT TIP
You can also use the goblet squat as a hip, ankle and knee mobility exercise by warming up with a light weight, and holding at the bottom of the move.

Stand with your feet shoulder-width apart holding a dumbbell or kettlebell like a drinking goblet. Keeping your core braced, squat until you can touch your knees with your elbows. Drive up through your heels to return to the start position.

Holding a dumbbell in each hand, step up onto a box set at knee height. Aim to push off your leading leg, without using your trailing leg (to help reinforce good form, raise the toes on your rear foot before moving). Step back down again.

 HANGING LEG RAISE

SETS 3 REPS 12 TEMPO 2111 REST 10sec

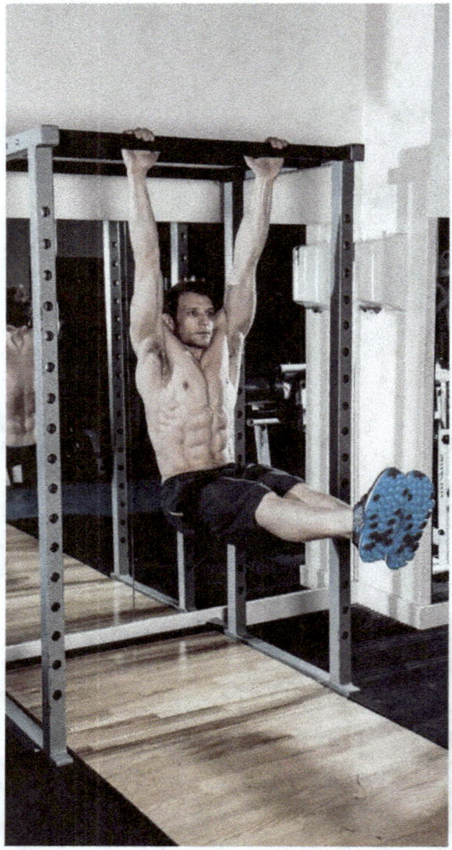

Hang from a bar and bring your legs up until they are parallel to the floor, using your lower abs to finish the movement without swinging your legs. If grip's a factor, you can use hanging slings.

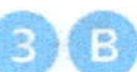 MED BALL KNEE RAISE

SETS 3 REPS 12 TEMPO 2111 REST 45sec

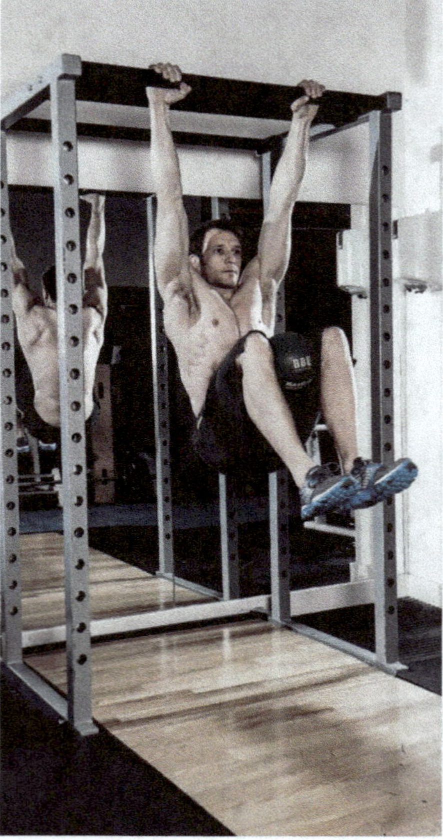

Hanging from a bar, hold a medicine ball between your knees. Bring your knees up until your thighs are at roughly 45° to your torso. Lower back to the start under control.

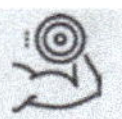

WORKOUT 3

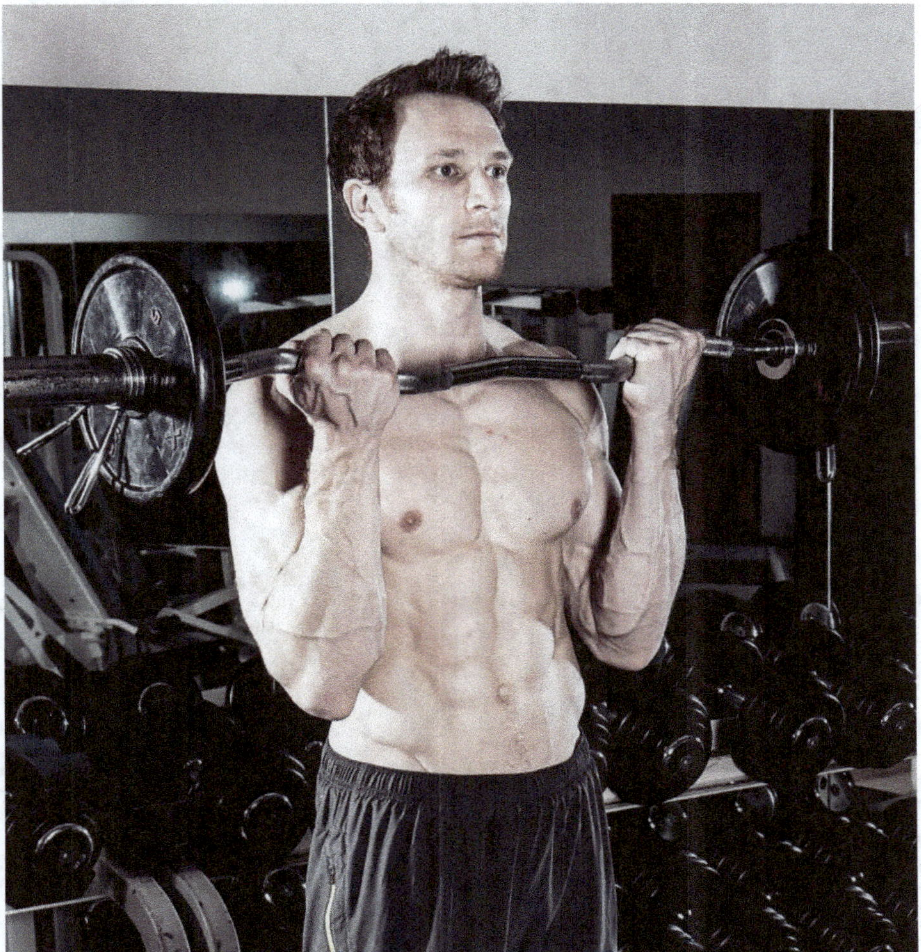

1 A CHIN-UP

SETS 5 REPS 6–10 TEMPO 2010 REST 10sec

1 B TRICEPS DIP

SETS 5 REPS 8 TEMPO 2010 REST 45sec

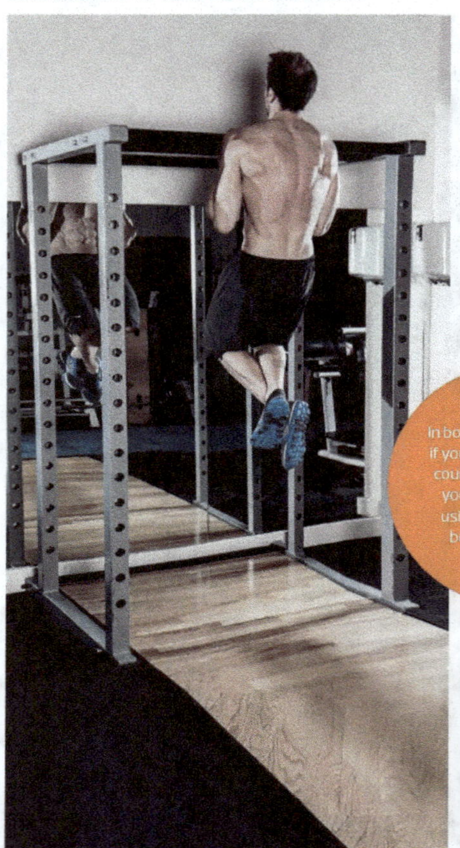

Hang from a bar with your palms facing towards you, shoulder blades retracted. Pull yourself up until your chin is above the bar, pause, then lower until your arms are straight again.

Grip a set of dip bars with your hands roughly shoulder-width apart, arms straight. Lower yourself until your upper arms are parallel to the floor, keeping your chest upright to hit your triceps. Press back up.

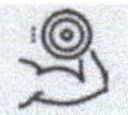

WORKOUT 3

2 A EZ-BAR BICEPS CURL

SETS 4 **REPS** 10 **TEMPO** 2010 **REST** 10sec

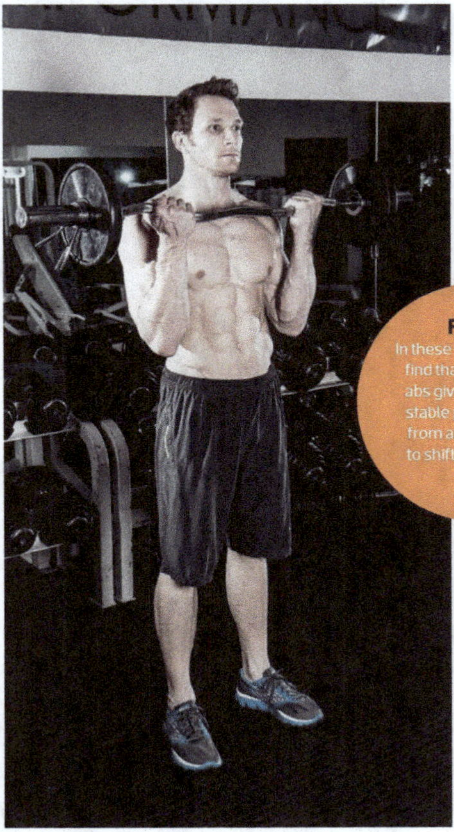

Using an EZ-bar reduces stress on your elbows. Stand straight and curl the bar upwards. Squeeze your biceps at the top of the movement and your triceps at the bottom.

2 B EZ-BAR TRICEPS EXTENSION

SETS 4 **REPS** 10 **TEMPO** 2010 **REST** 45sec

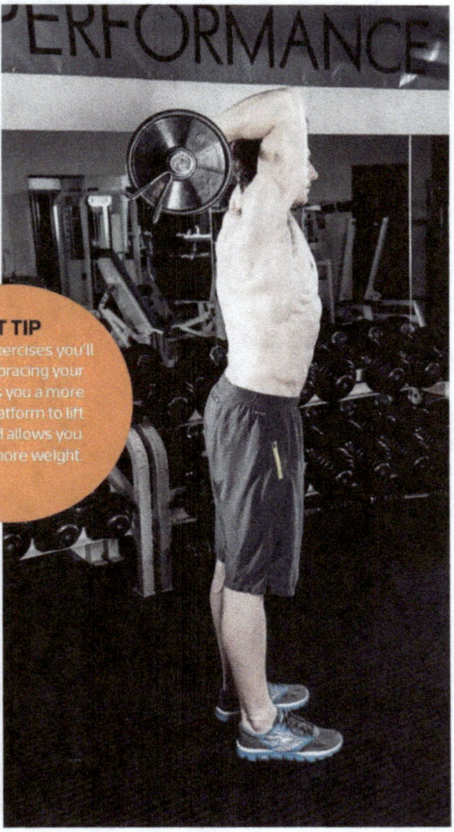

FIT TIP
In these exercises you'll find that bracing your abs gives you a more stable platform to lift from and allows you to shift more weight.

Stand holding an EZ-bar above your head, palms facing behind you. Lower the bar behind your head by bending your elbows. Pause, and then lift the weight by contracting your triceps.

3 A CABLE HAMMER CURL

SETS 3 REPS 12 TEMPO 2111 REST 10sec

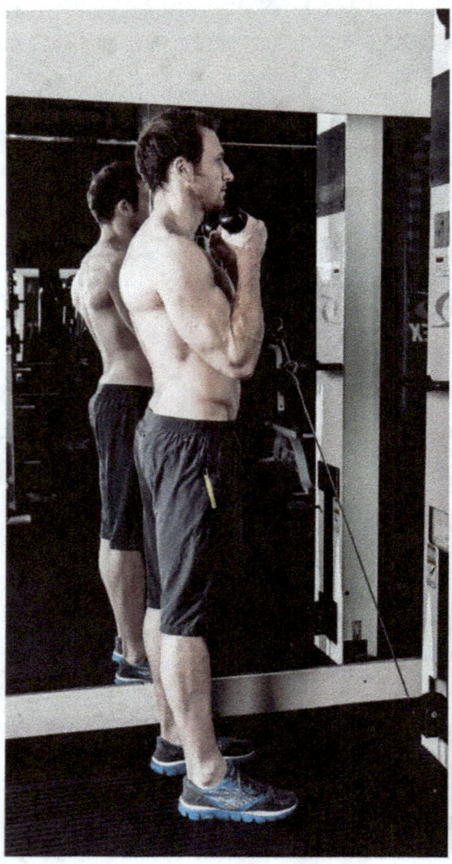

Holding a cable rope attachment in both hands, curl it upwards towards your chest, pause and then lower. Keep the tension on the cable throughout the move, and avoid using momentum.

3 B CABLE PRESS-DOWN

SETS 3 REPS 12 TEMPO 2111 REST 45sec

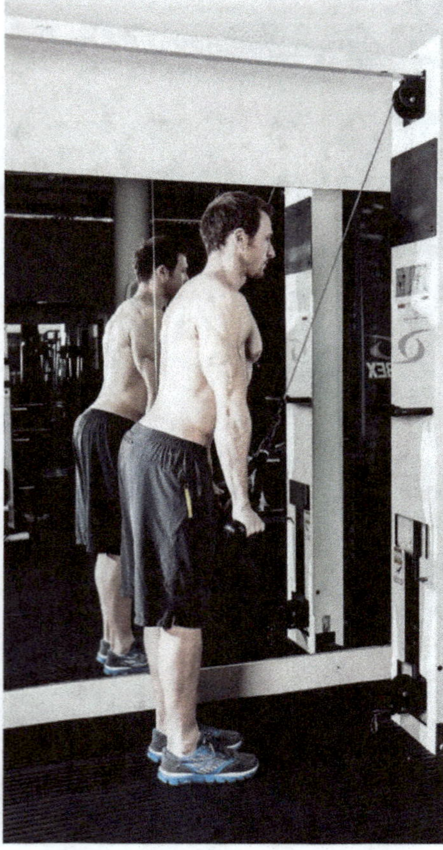

Still holding the cable rope attachment, press down on the ropes to lift the stack, squeezing your triceps at the end of the movement. Avoid using the rest of your body to shift the weight.

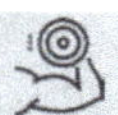

WORKOUT 4

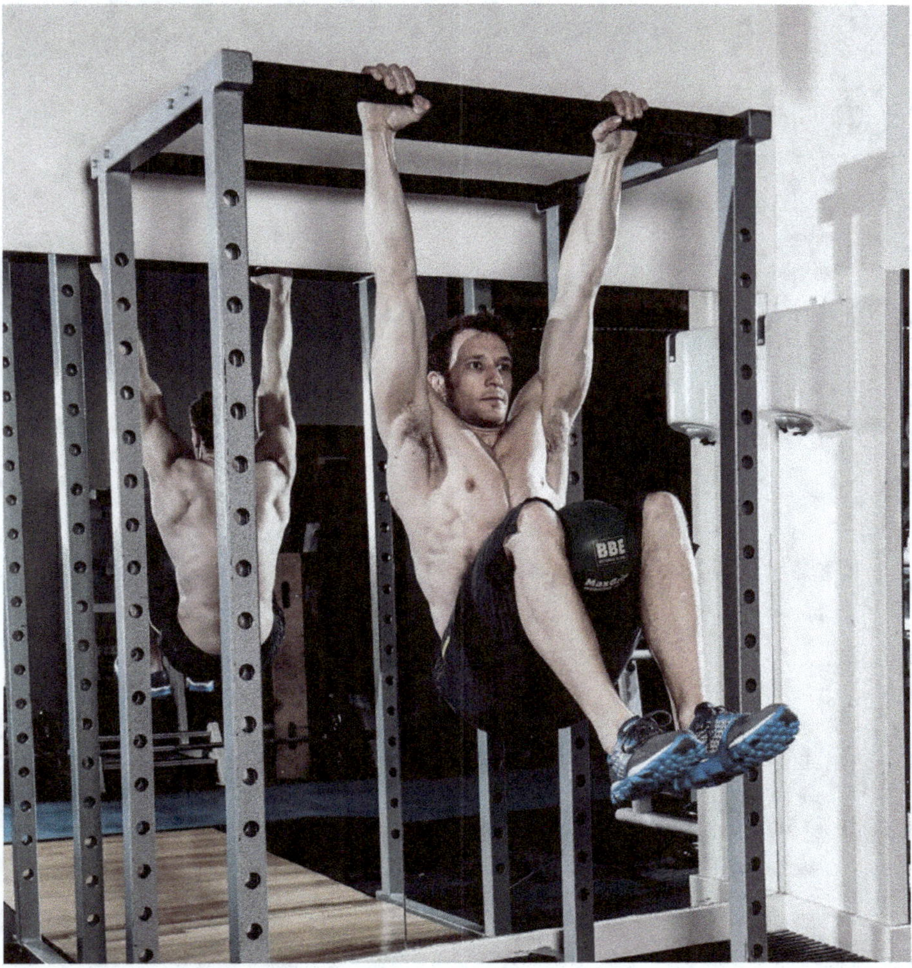

1 A OVERHEAD PRESS

SETS 5 **REPS** 8 **TEMPO** 2010 **REST** 10sec

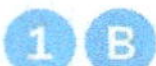

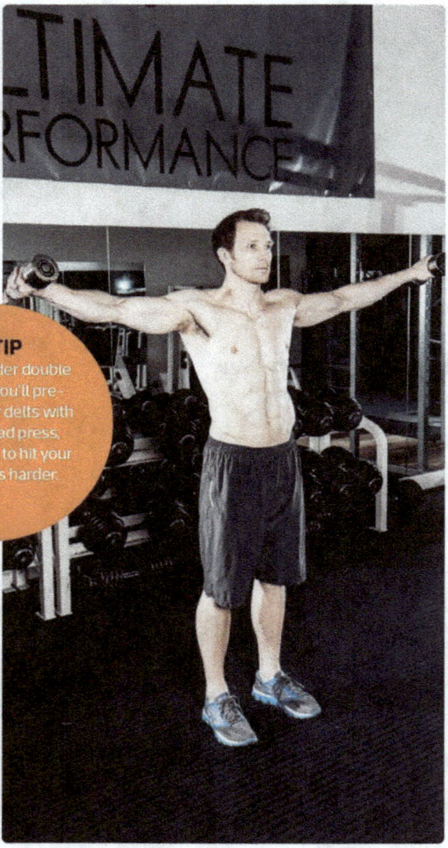

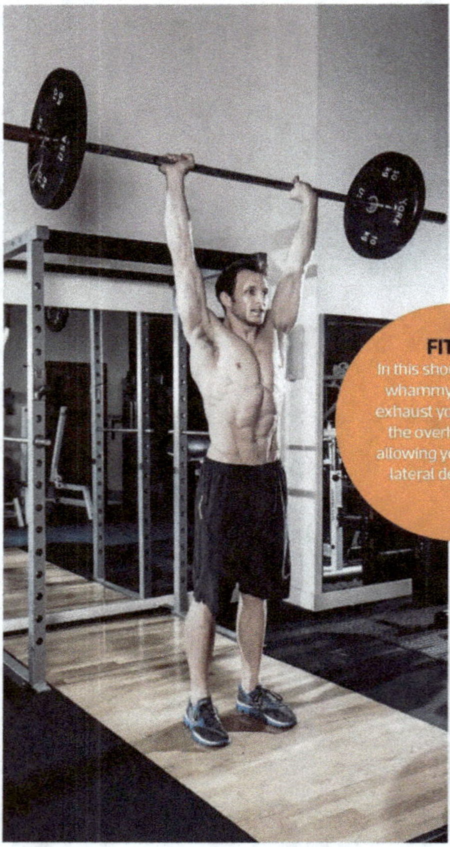

Hold the bar with your thumbs wrapped on the same side as your fingers, touching your shoulders. Brace your glutes and core and press the bar overhead, putting your head through the 'window' of your arms at the top. Lower under control.

1 B DB LATERAL RAISE

SETS 5 **REPS** 8 **TEMPO** 2010 **REST** 45sec

FIT TIP
In this shoulder double whammy, you'll pre-exhaust your delts with the overhead press, allowing you to hit your lateral delts harder.

Hold a light dumbbell in each hand. Raise them out to the sides, keeping a slight bend in your elbows. To keep the tension on the right muscles, keep your pinkies higher than your thumbs and don't go above shoulder height.

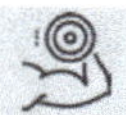

WORKOUT 4

2 A DB UPRIGHT ROW

SETS 4 REPS 10 TEMPO 2010 REST 10sec

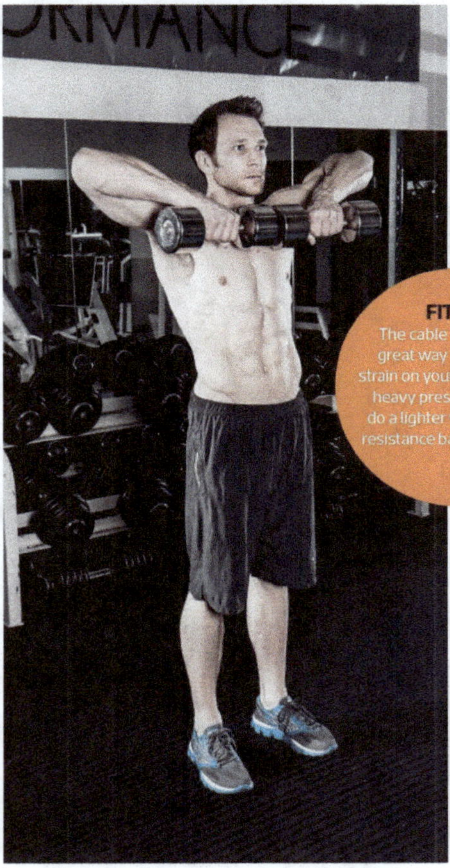

2 B CABLE FACE PULL

SETS 4 REPS 10 TEMPO 2010 REST 45sec

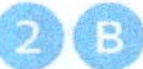

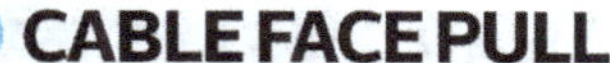

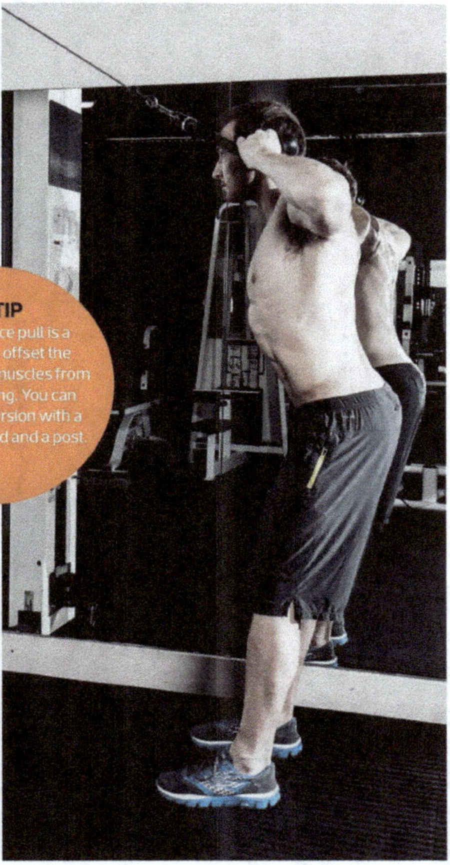

FIT TIP
The cable face pull is a great way to offset the strain on your muscles from heavy pressing. You can do a lighter version with a resistance band and a post.

Hold a dumbbell in each hand. Pull them up to the top of your chest, bringing your elbows out to the sides. Avoid jerking or using momentum to safeguard your rotator cuffs. Lower under control.

Hold the handles of a cable rope attachment with your palms facing downward and the cable set at head height. Pull the rope handles to either side of your forehead, pulling your elbows behind you.

  HANGING LEG RAISE

SETS 3 REPS 12 TEMPO 2111 REST 10sec

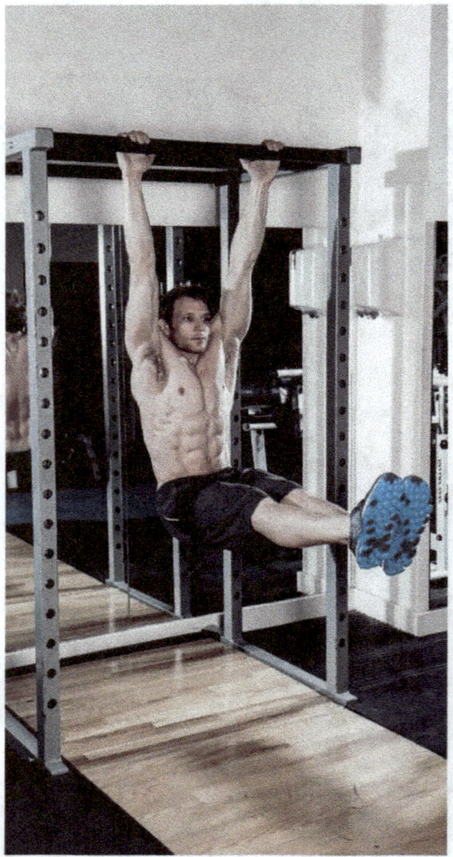

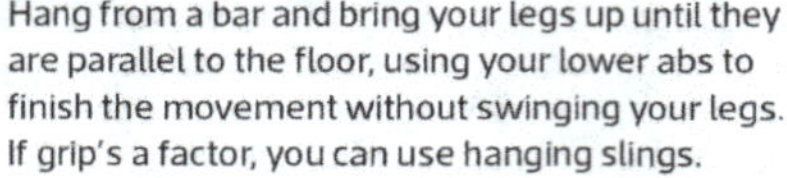

Hang from a bar and bring your legs up until they are parallel to the floor, using your lower abs to finish the movement without swinging your legs. If grip's a factor, you can use hanging slings.

 MED BALL KNEE RAISE

SETS 3 REPS 12 TEMPO 2111 REST 45sec

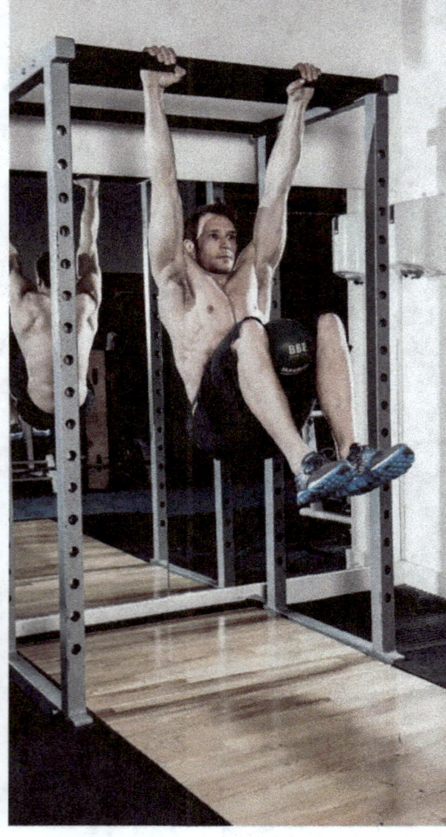

Hanging from a bar, hold a medicine ball between your knees. Bring your knees up until your thighs are at roughly 45° to your torso. Lower back to the start under control.

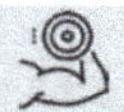

WEEK 2

Once again, the moves stay the same but the volume is increased

WORKOUT 1 **CHEST AND BACK**

EXERCISE	SETS	REPS	TEMPO	REST
1A Incline dumbbell bench press	5	10	2010	10SEC
1B Dumbbell one-arm bent-over row	5	10 EACH SIDE	2111	45SEC
2A Cable cross-over	4	12	2111	10SEC
2B Lat pull-down	4	12	2111	45SEC
3A Cable flye	3	15	2111	10SEC
3B Bent-over reverse flye	3	15	2111	45SEC

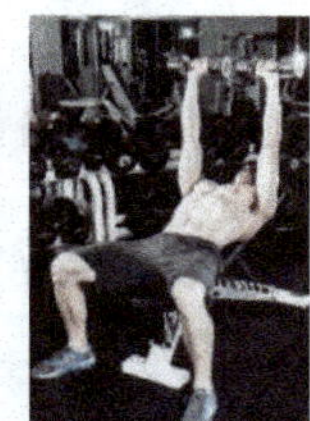

WORKOUT 2 **LEGS AND CORE**

EXERCISE	SETS	REPS	TEMPO	REST
1A Barbell lunge	5	10 EACH SIDE	2010	10SEC
1B Leg press	5	10	2010	45SEC
2A Goblet squat	4	12	2010	10SEC
2B Dumbbell step-up	4	12 EACH SIDE	1010	45SEC
3A Hanging leg raise	3	15	1111	10SEC
3B Medicine ball knee raise	3	15	1111	45SEC

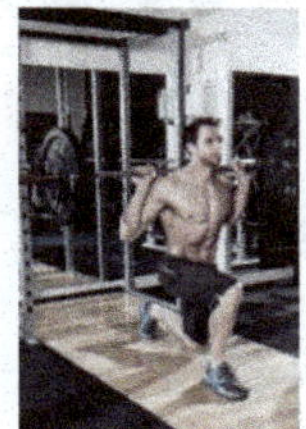

WORKOUT 3 **BICEPS AND TRICEPS**

EXERCISE	SETS	REPS	TEMPO	REST
1A Chin-up	5	10	2111	10SEC
1B Triceps dip	5	10	2010	45SEC
2A EZ-bar biceps curl	4	12	2111	10SEC
2B Standing EZ-bar triceps extension	4	12	2010	45SEC
3A Cable rope hammer curl	3	15	2111	10SEC
3B Cable rope triceps press-down	3	15	2010	45SEC

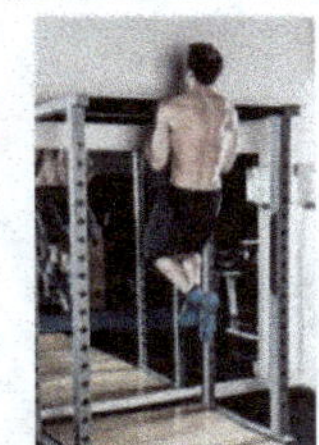

WORKOUT 4 **SHOULDERS AND CORE**

EXERCISE	SETS	REPS	TEMPO	REST
1A Overhead press	5	10	2010	10SEC
1B Dumbbell lateral raise	5	10	1110	45SEC
2A Dumbbell upright row	4	12	2111	10SEC
2B Cable face pull	4	12	1110	45SEC
3A Hanging leg raise	3	15	2110	10SEC
3B Medicine ball knee raise	3	15	1110	45SEC

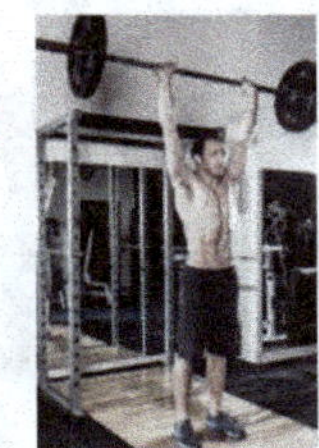

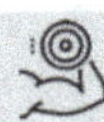

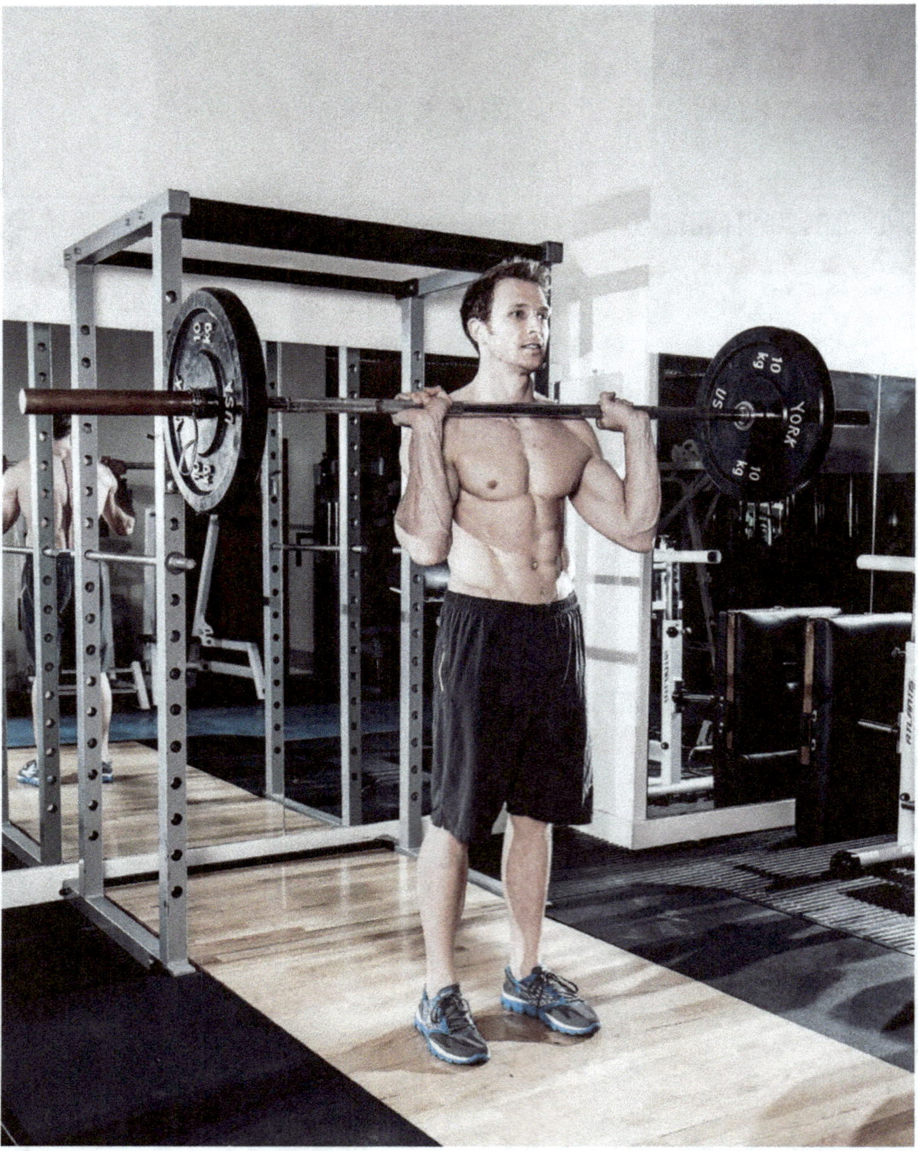

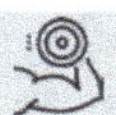

WEEK 3 WORKOUT 1

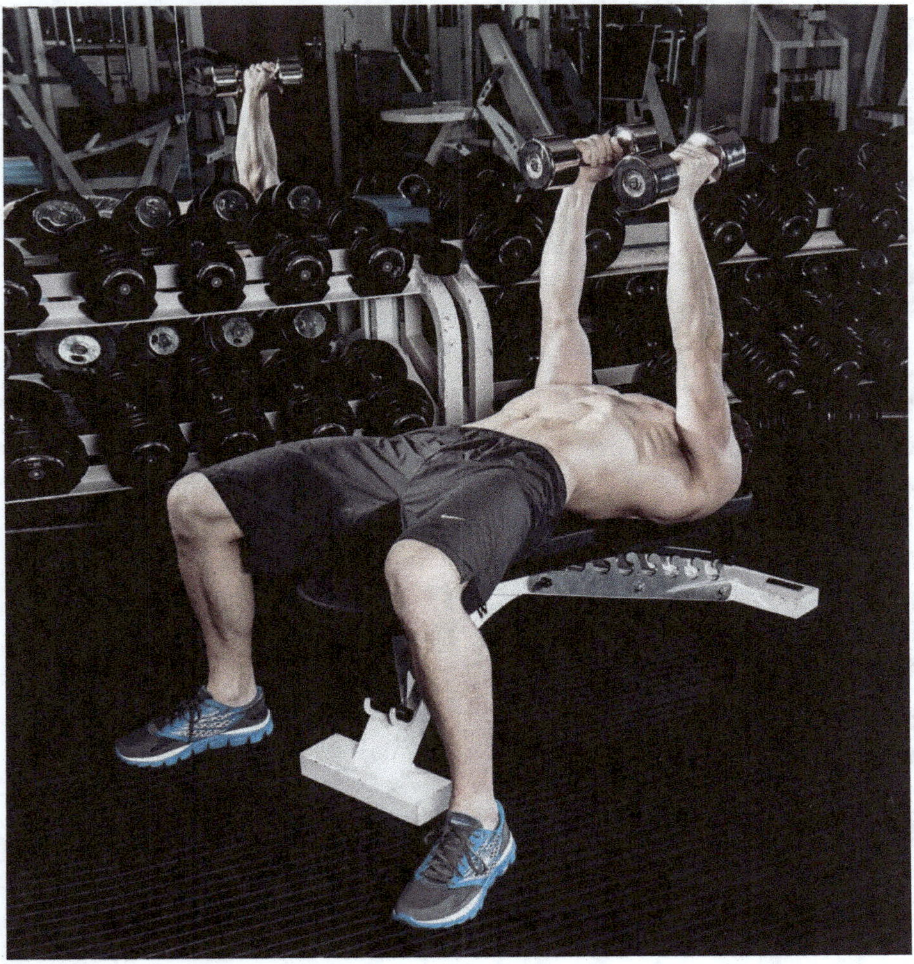

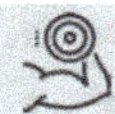

1 A INCLINE BENCH PRESS

SETS 5 **REPS** 8 **TEMPO** 2010 **REST** 10sec

1 B WIDE-GRIP SEATED ROW

SETS 5 **REPS** 8 **TEMPO** 2110 **REST** 45sec

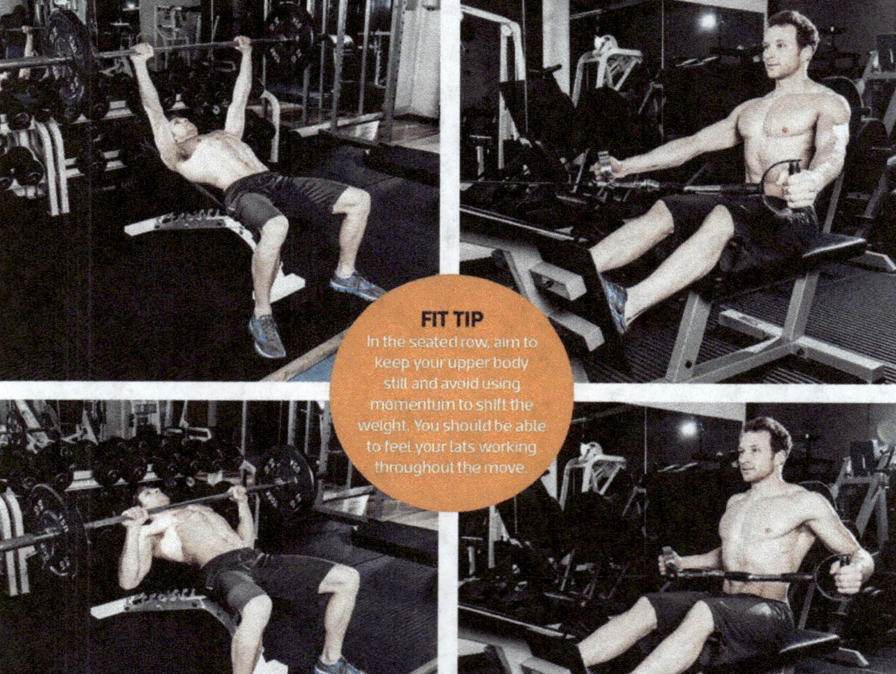

Lie on an incline bench with your feet on the floor. Hold the bar with an overhand grip with your hands shoulder-width apart. Slowly lower the bar to your chest, then drive it strongly upwards.

Sit on the machine with a wide-grip attachment, knees slightly bent. Pull the handle in to your sternum, bringing your elbows behind you and your shoulder blades together. Pause, then return to the start position.

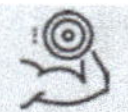

WORKOUT 1

② Ⓐ LYING DB PULL-OVER

SETS 4 REPS 10 TEMPO 1110 REST 10sec

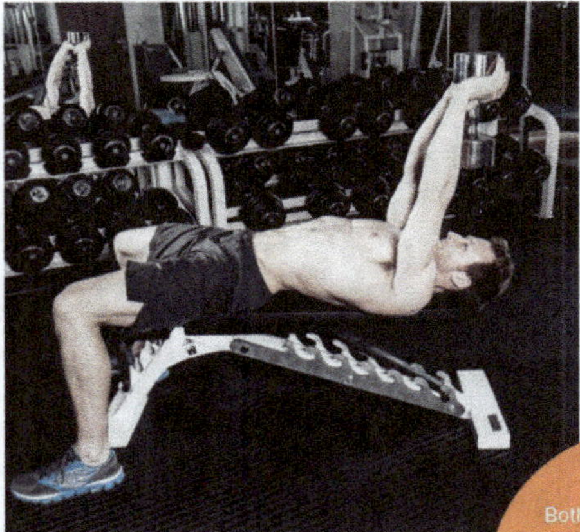

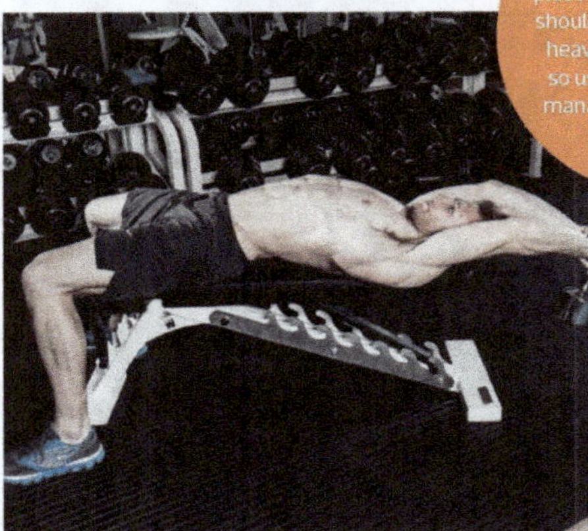

Lie on a bench with a dumbbell in both hands, directly above your head. Let the dumbbell descend behind your head, with your arms fairly straight. Pause, then 'pull' it back up to the start position.

② Ⓑ LYING DB FLYE

SETS 4 REPS 10 TEMPO 1110 REST 45sec

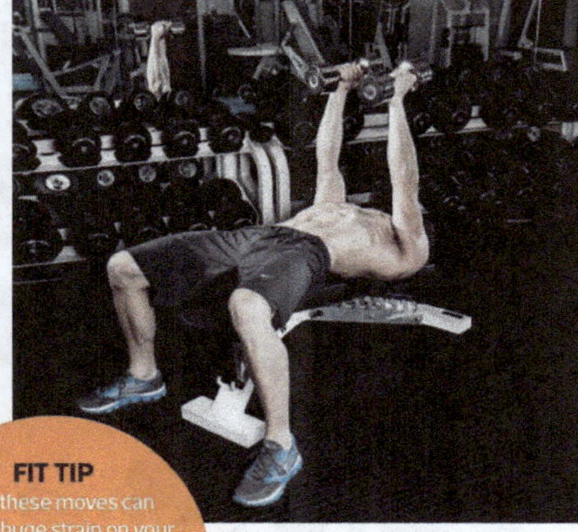

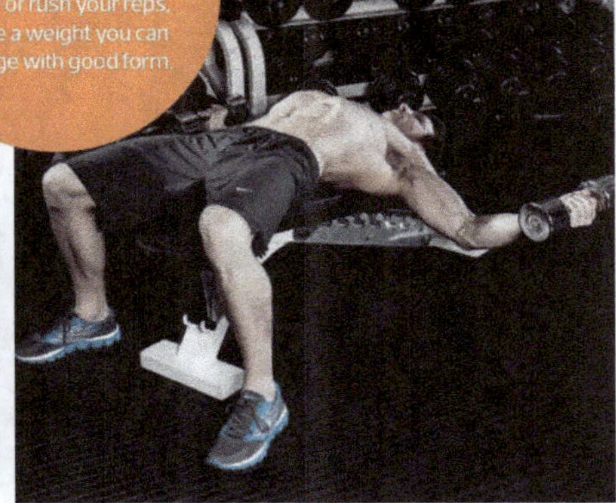

FIT TIP
Both these moves can place a huge strain on your shoulder joint if you go too heavy or rush your reps, so use a weight you can manage with good form.

Lie on a bench with the dumbbells above you, palms facing in. Bring your arms apart, keeping your elbows slightly bent, until you feel the stretch in your chest, then bring them back together.

3 A WIDE-GRIP PULL-DOWN

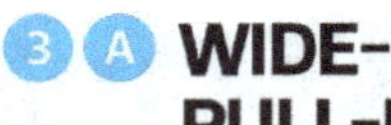

SETS 3 REPS 12 TEMPO 2010 REST 10sec

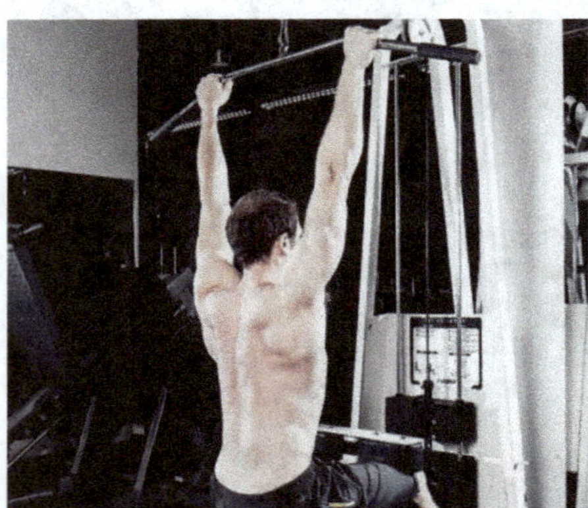

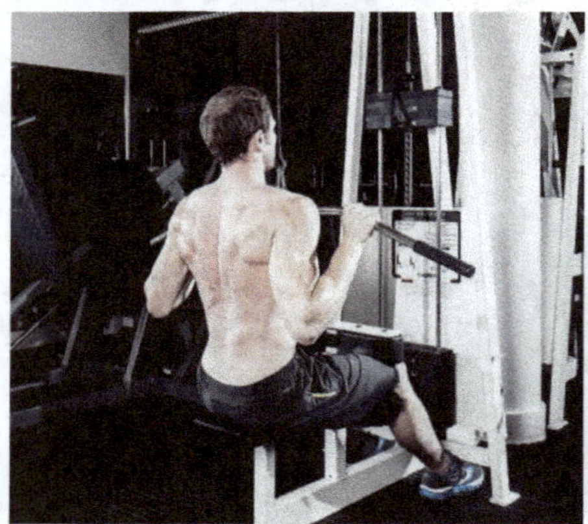

Sit on the pull-down machine and take a wide grip on the bar, hands almost double shoulder-width apart. Pull the bar down to your chest, aiming to bring your elbows behind you. Focus on keeping your shoulder blades engaged.

3 B CABLE CROSS-OVER

SETS 3 REPS 12 TEMPO 2010 REST 45sec

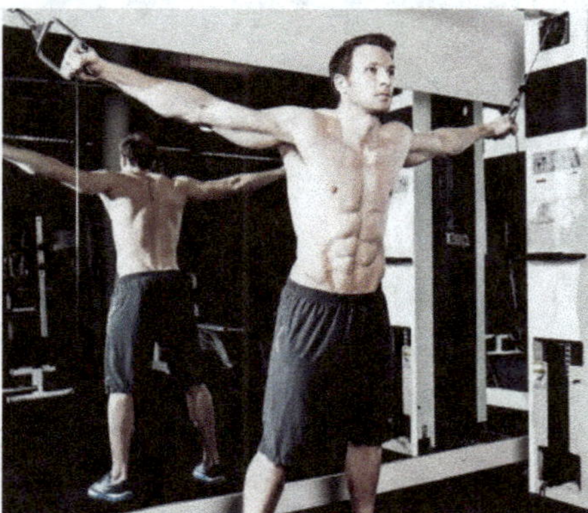

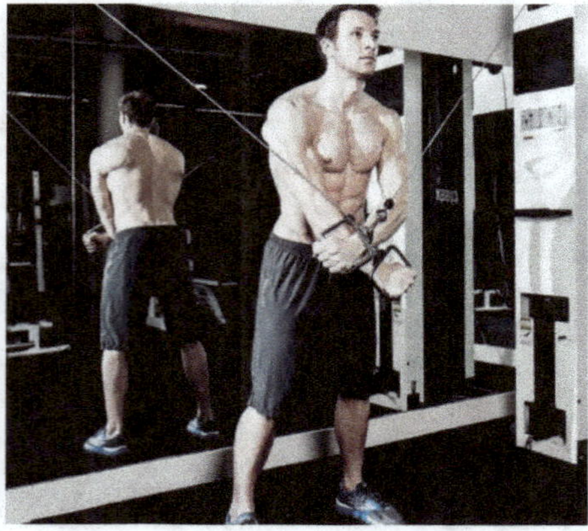

Stand with a split stance holding a D-handle attachment in each hand, with the cable set above shoulder height. Bring your hands down in an arc to meet in front of your chest, squeeze your chest muscles, then return to the start.

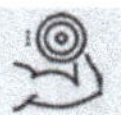

WORKOUT 2

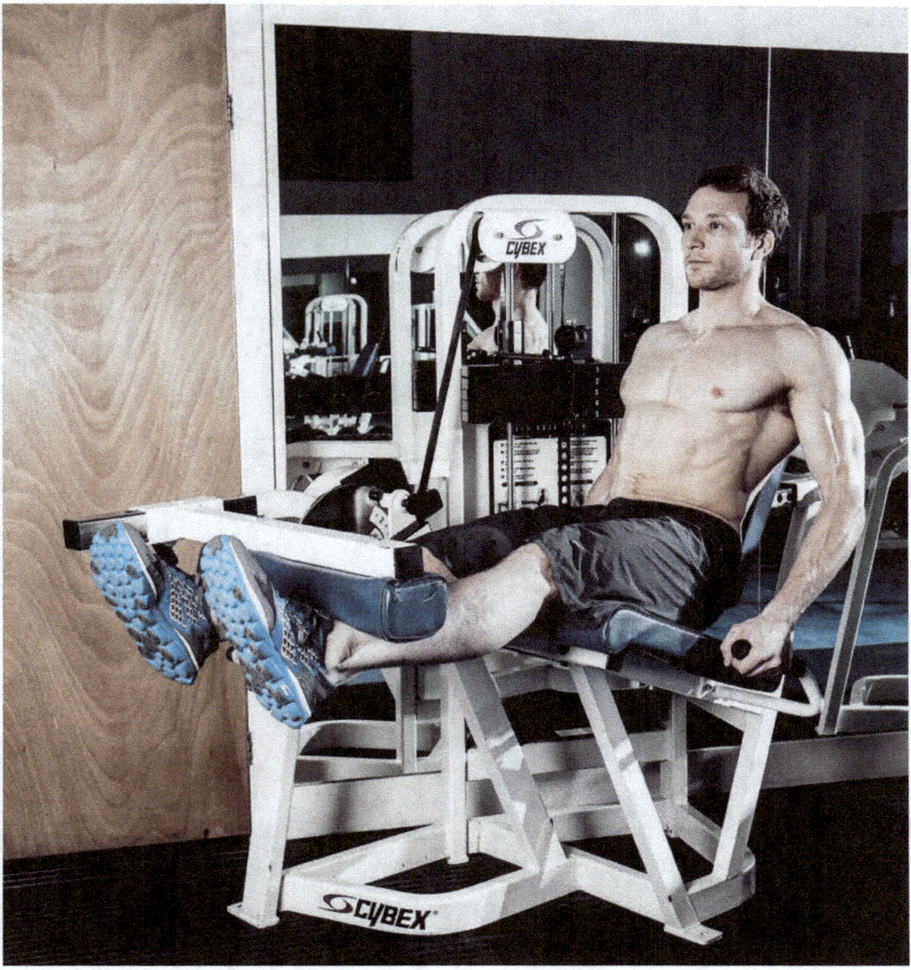

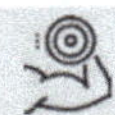

1 A DEADLIFT

SETS 5 REPS 8 TEMPO 2010 REST 10sec

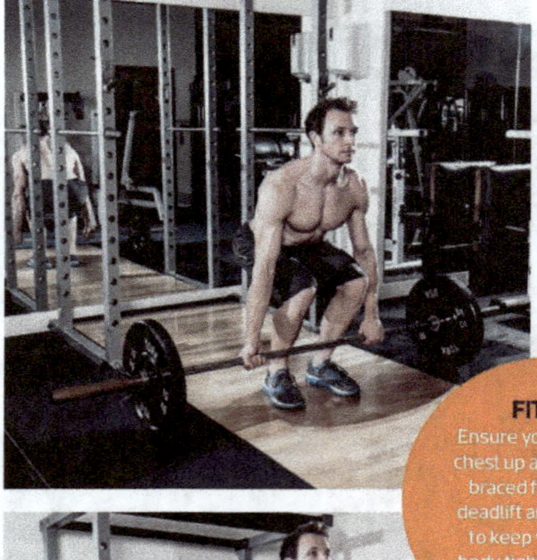

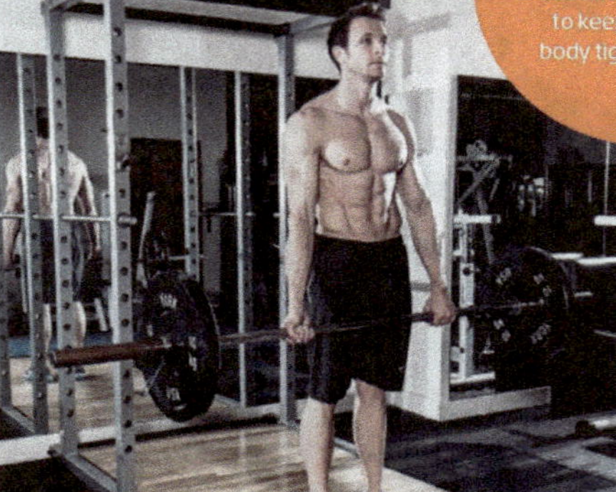

Stand with your toes under the bar, feet hip-width apart. Grab the bar with your arms vertical and just outside your knees. Straighten your back by raising your chest and driving your hips forward, pulling the bar against your shins.

1 B BB SQUAT

SETS 5 REPS 8 TEMPO 2010 REST 45sec

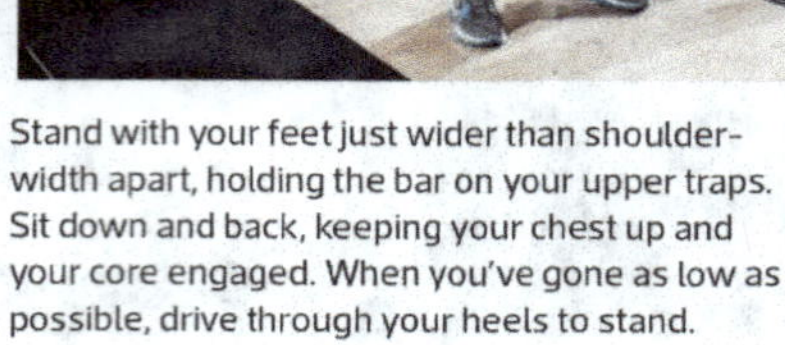

FIT TIP
Ensure you keep your chest up and your core braced for both the deadlift and the squat to keep your upper body tight and stable.

Stand with your feet just wider than shoulder-width apart, holding the bar on your upper traps. Sit down and back, keeping your chest up and your core engaged. When you've gone as low as possible, drive through your heels to stand.

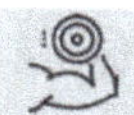

WORKOUT 2

2 A LEG EXTENSION

SETS 4 REPS 10 TEMPO 1110 REST 10sec

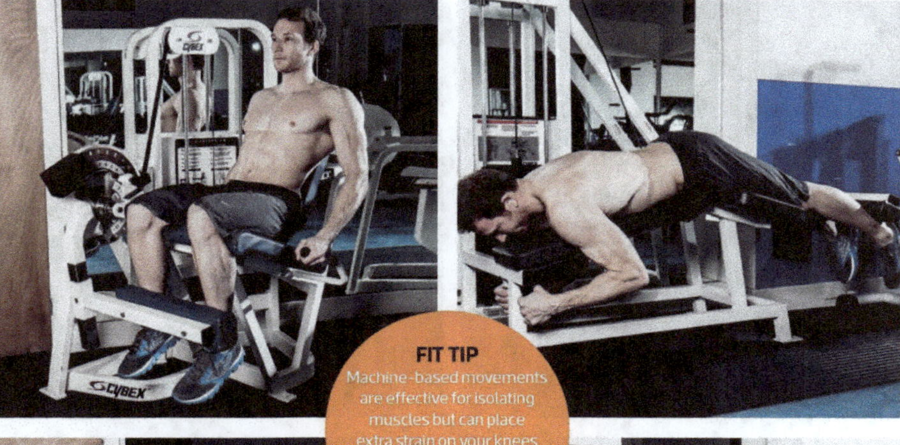

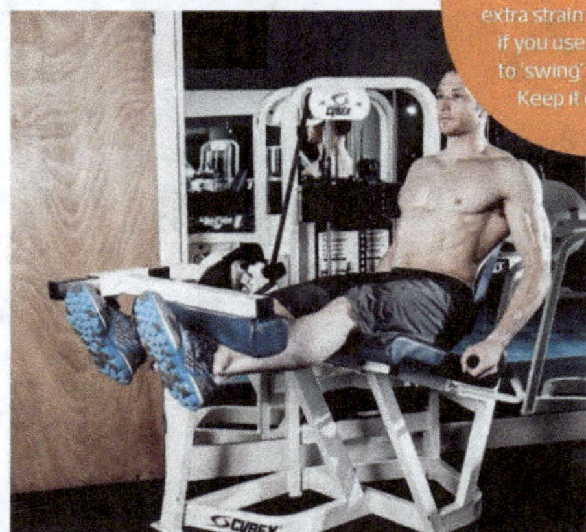

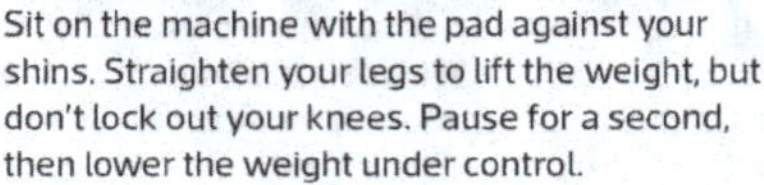

2 B LEG CURL

SETS 4 REPS 10 TEMPO 1110 REST 45sec

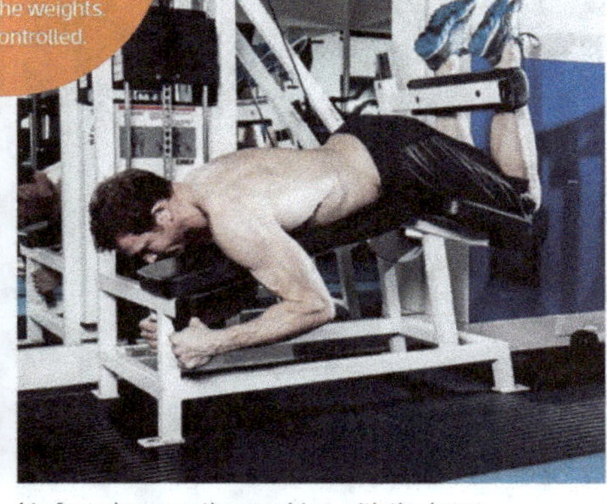

FIT TIP
Machine-based movements are effective for isolating muscles but can place extra strain on your knees if you use momentum to 'swing' the weights. Keep it controlled.

Sit on the machine with the pad against your shins. Straighten your legs to lift the weight, but don't lock out your knees. Pause for a second, then lower the weight under control.

Lie face down on the machine with the lever adjusted to fit your height (an angled machine is slightly better for hamstring recruitment). Curl up as far as possible without lifting your upper legs from the pad, pause and lower slowly.

 BICYCLE

SETS 3 REPS 12 TEMPO 2010 REST 10sec

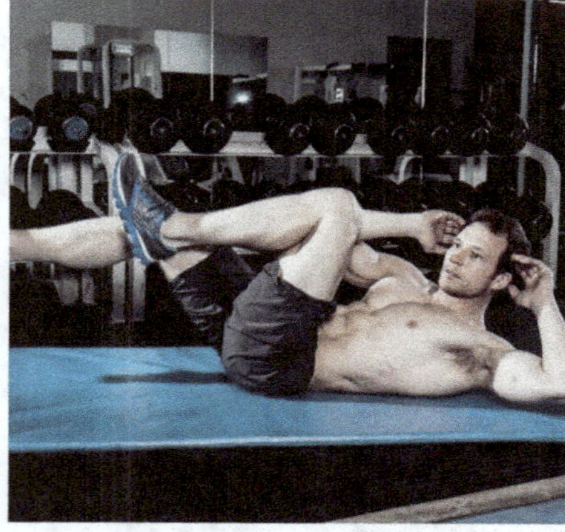

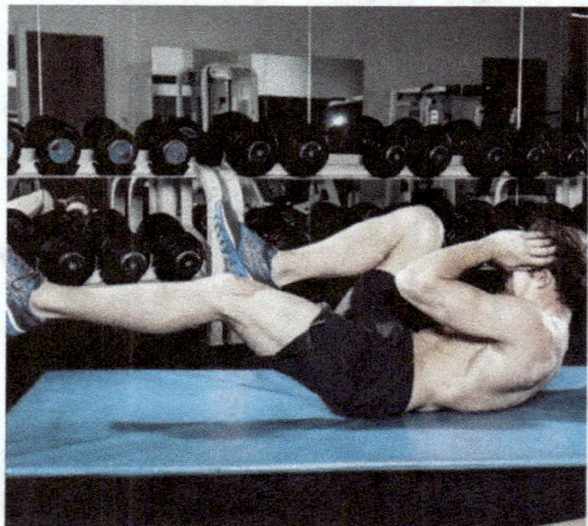

Lie on your back with your fingers touching –
not supporting – your head. Bring one elbow
to the opposite knee, then repeat on the other
side, keeping the movement controlled and
feeling the tension across your abs.

 OBLIQUE CRUNCH

SETS 3 REPS 12 TEMPO 2010 REST 45sec

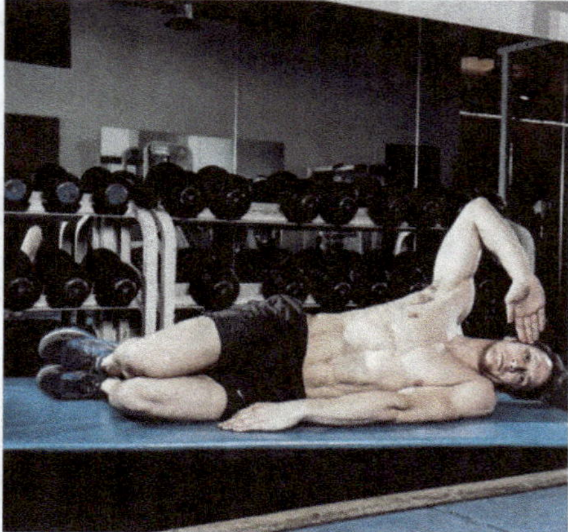

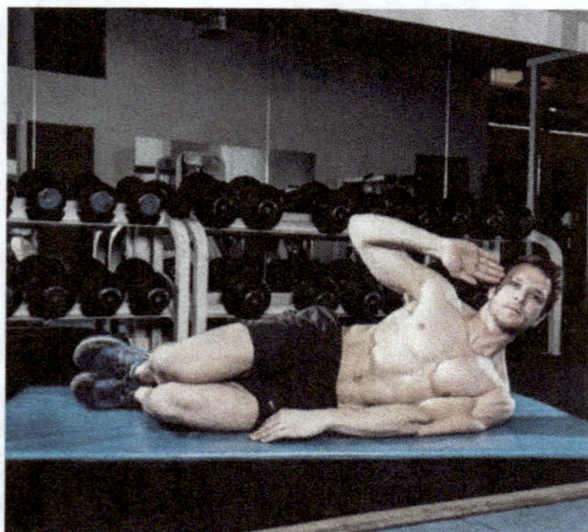

Lie on your side with your knees bent, then use
your obliques (side abs muscles) to raise your
torso off the floor. Pause at the top, squeeze
your abs, then lower back to the start.

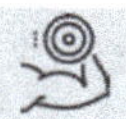

WORKOUT 3

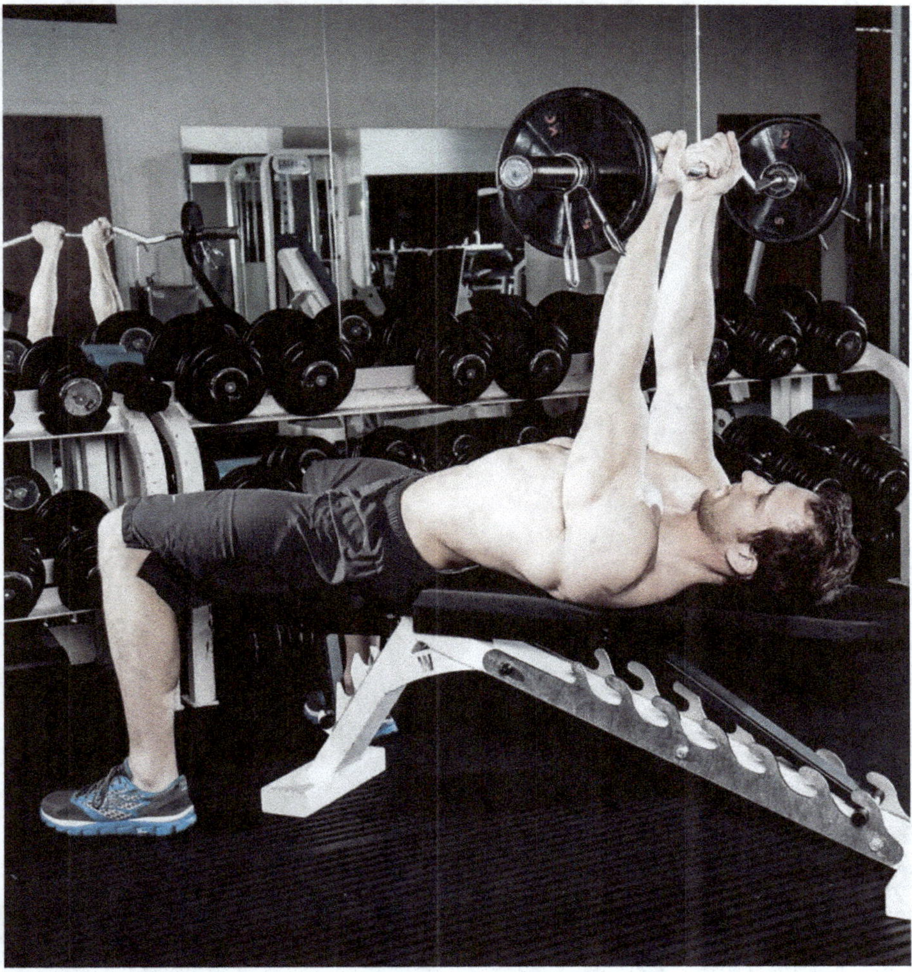

  WEIGHTED CHIN-UP

SETS 5 **REPS** 8 **TEMPO** 2010 **REST** 10sec

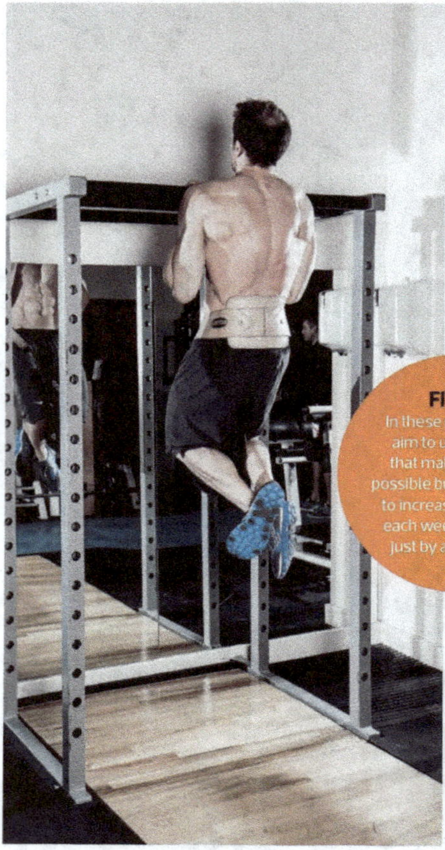

 WEIGHTED TRICEPS DIP

SETS 5 **REPS** 8 **TEMPO** 2010 **REST** 45sec

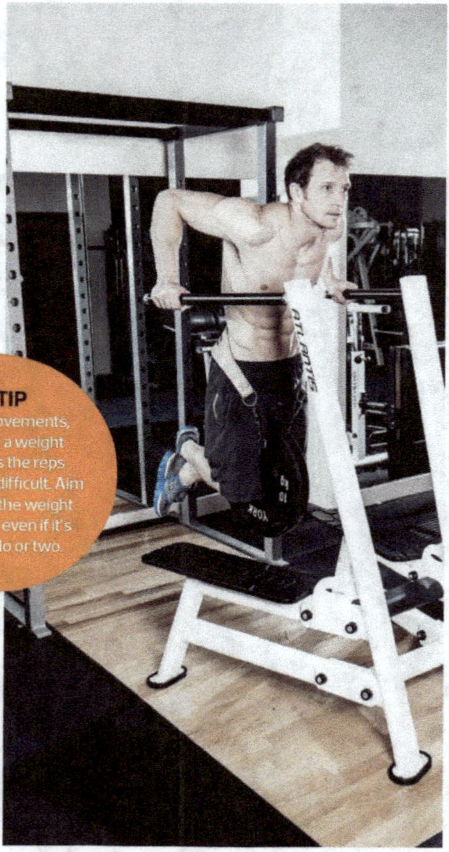

FIT TIP

In these movements, aim to use a weight that makes the reps possible but difficult. Aim to increase the weight each week, even if it's just by a kilo or two.

Wearing a weight belt or vest or holding a dumbbell between your feet, hang from a bar with palms facing you. Pull up until your chin's over the bar. Pause, then lower – don't drop, or you'll risk hurting your elbows at the bottom.

With a weight belt around your waist, grip a set of dip bars with your hands roughly shoulder-width apart, arms straight. Lower yourself until your upper arms are parallel to the floor, keeping your chest upright to hit your triceps. Press back up.

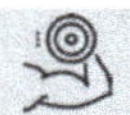

WORKOUT 3

  ## EZ-BAR PREACHER CURL

SETS 4 **REPS** 10 **TEMPO** 1110 **REST** 10sec

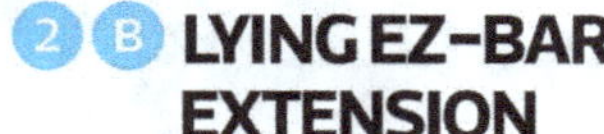 ## LYING EZ-BAR EXTENSION

SETS 4 **REPS** 10 **TEMPO** 1110 **REST** 45sec

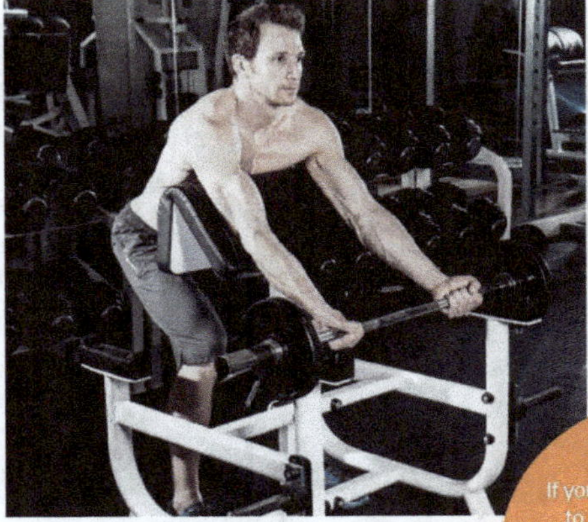

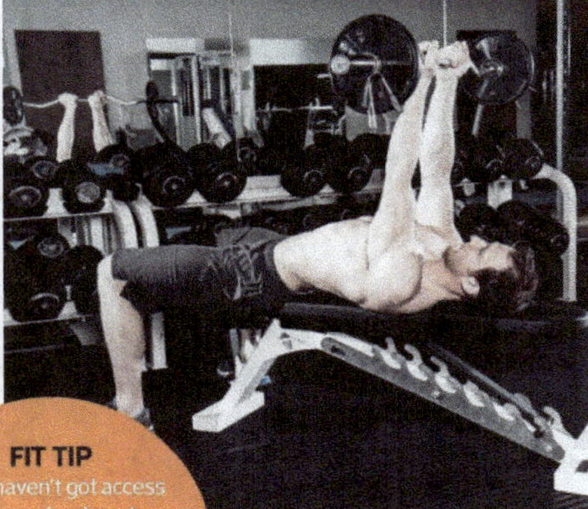

FIT TIP
If you haven't got access to a preacher bench, do single-arm curls with a normal bench at a high incline – it's less effective, but still works.

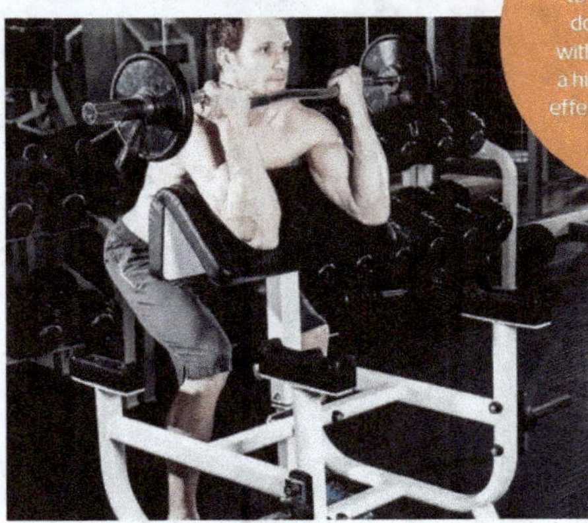

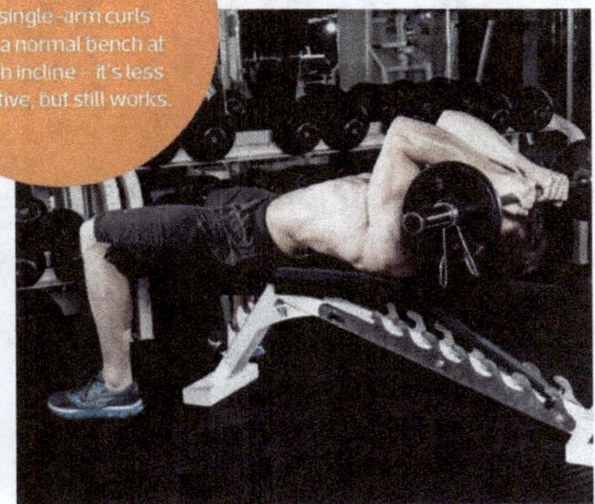

Sit at a preacher bench holding an EZ-bar with palms facing up. Curl the bar up to your chin, squeeze your biceps at the top, then lower it under control. Keep your elbows locked in position, avoiding using momentum to finish the move.

Lie on a bench, holding an EZ-bar above your chest with straight arms. Slowly lower the bar towards the top of your head by bending your elbows, which should stay pointing directly to the ceiling. Then straighten your arms.

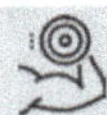

  SPIDER CURL

SETS 3 REPS 12 TEMPO 2010 REST 10sec

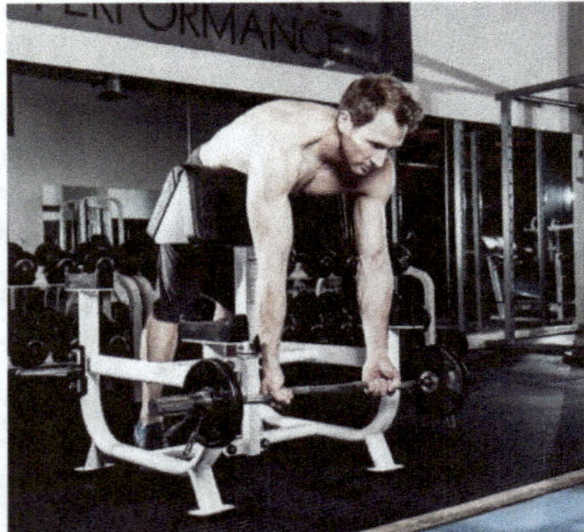

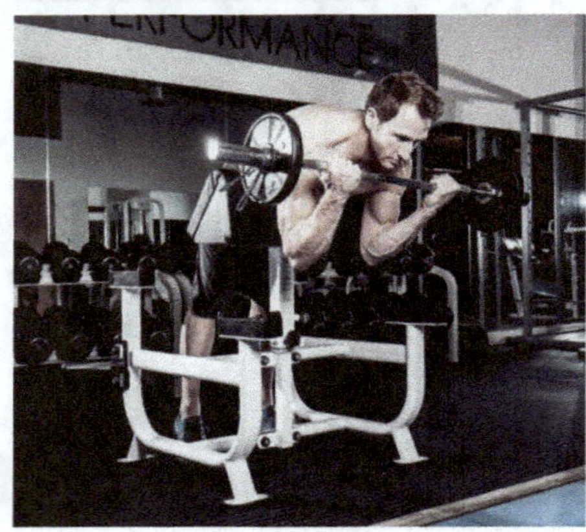

Lean over a preacher bench holding a bar so that your arms hang straight down, then curl the bar upwards. You'll benefit from an increased range of motion while still keeping your upper body supported.

 CABLE EXTENSION

SETS 3 REPS 12 TEMPO 2010 REST 45sec

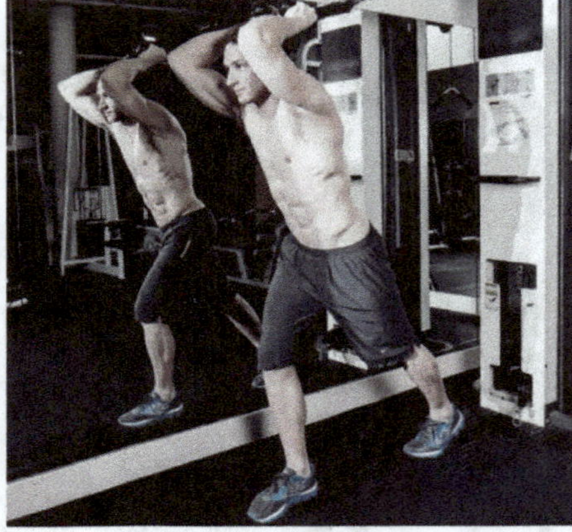

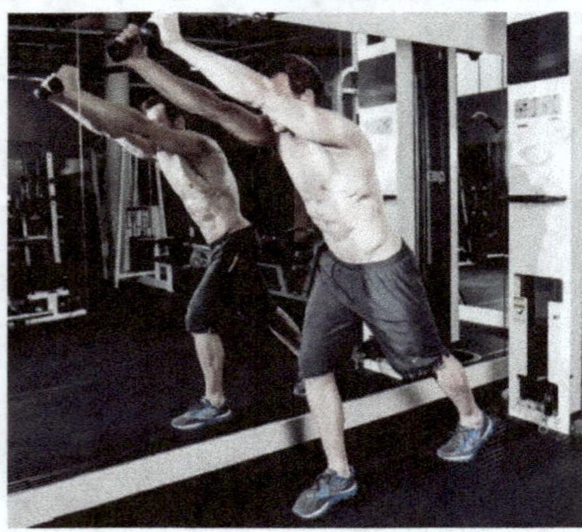

Stand facing away from a cable machine, holding the handles of a rope attachment with your arms bent behind your head. Extend your arms straight overhead, pause, then lower back to the start under control.

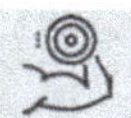

WORKOUT 4

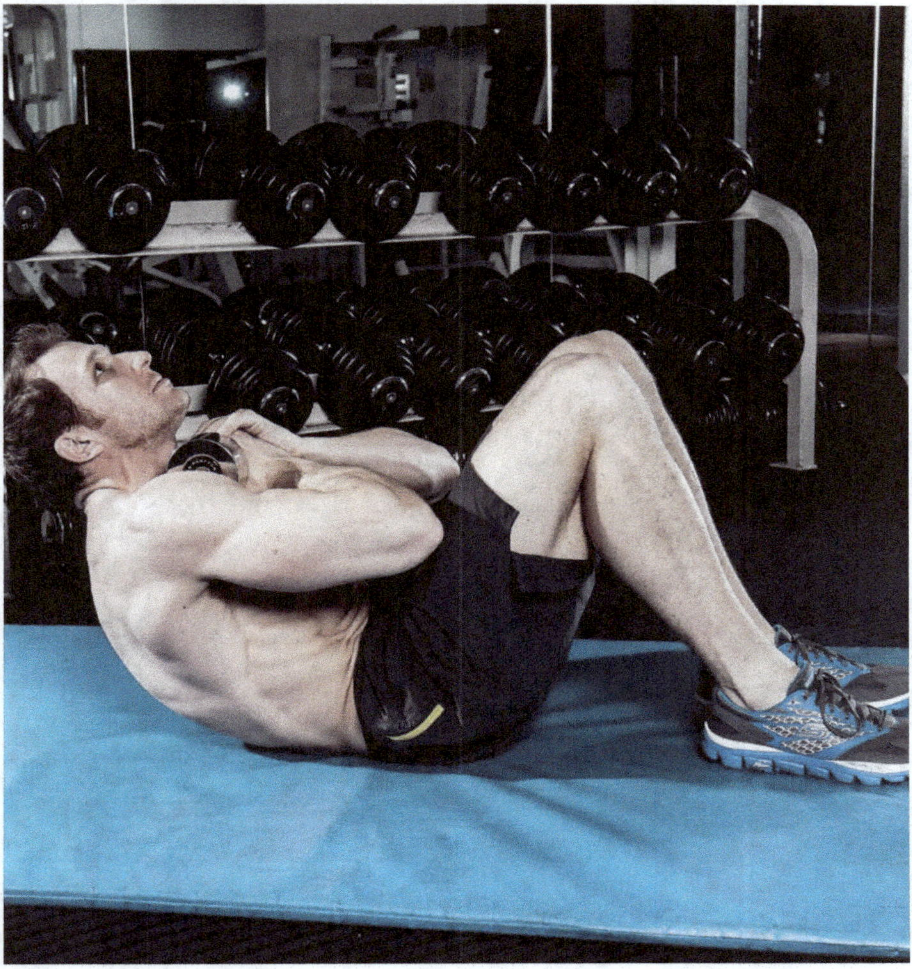

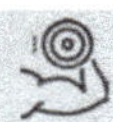

① Ⓐ PUSH PRESS

SETS 5 REPS 8 TEMPO 2010 REST 10sec

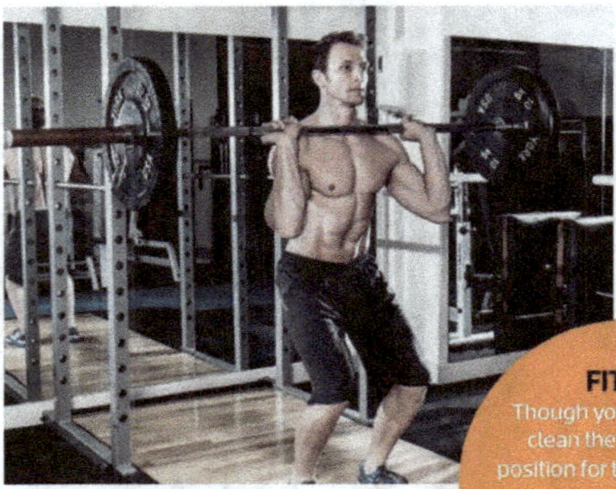

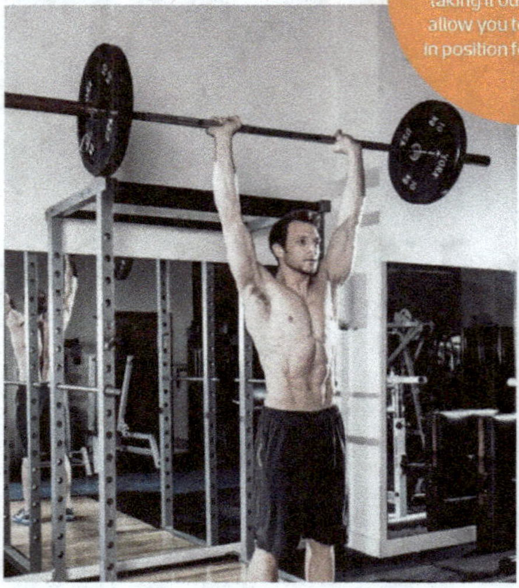

① Ⓑ EZ-BAR UPRIGHT ROW

SETS 5 REPS 8 TEMPO 2010 REST 45sec

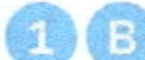

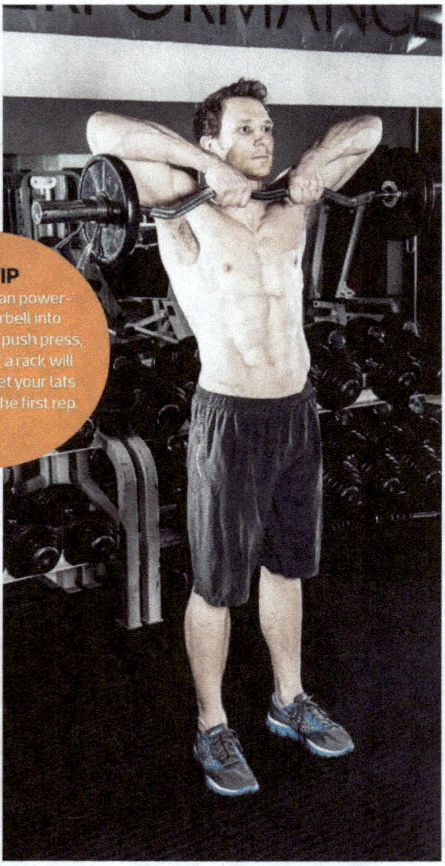

FIT TIP
Though you can power-clean the barbell into position for the push press, taking it out of a rack will allow you to set your lats in position for the first rep.

Hold the bar at shoulder level. Do a quarter-squat to gather momentum, then drive explosively through your heels to help you press the bar overhead. Pause at the top, and lower under control.

Hold an EZ-bar with your hands fairly close, palms facing you. Pull the bar up, bringing your elbows out to the sides, until it's under your chin. Pause, then lower. Don't use momentum - it's bad for your shoulders.

WORKOUT 4

② Ⓐ CABLE LATERAL RAISE

SETS 4 **REPS** 10 each side **TEMPO** 1110 **REST** 10sec

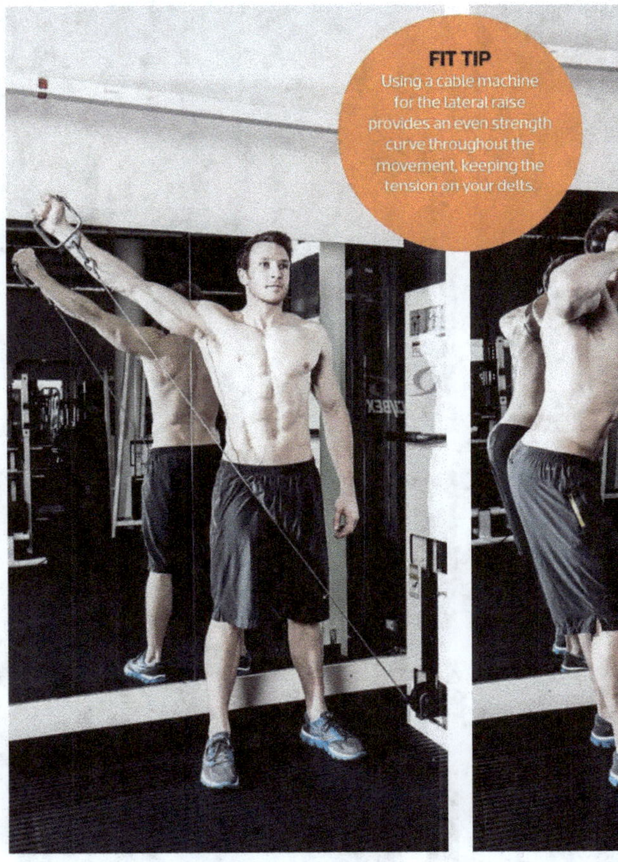

FIT TIP
Using a cable machine for the lateral raise provides an even strength curve throughout the movement, keeping the tension on your delts.

Stand side-on to a cable machine. Grasp the low attachment with the hand furthest away. Bring the cable up in a lateral movement, pause at shoulder height, then reverse the movement. Complete all the reps on one side, then switch.

② Ⓑ CABLE FACE PULL

SETS 4 **REPS** 10 **TEMPO** 1110 **REST** 45sec

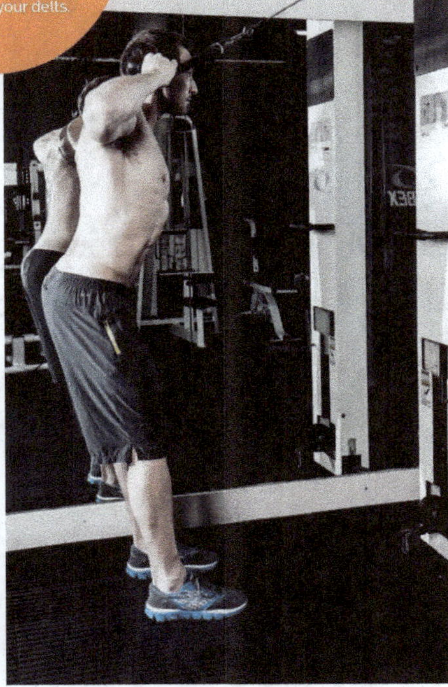

Hold the handles of a cable rope attachment with your palms facing downward and the cable set at head height. Pull the rope handles to either side of your forehead, pulling your elbows behind you.

3 A WEIGHTED CRUNCH

SETS 3 **REPS** 12 **TEMPO** 2010 **REST** 10sec

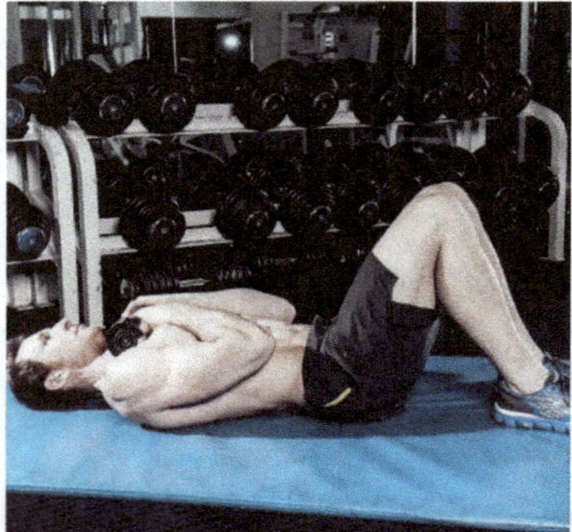

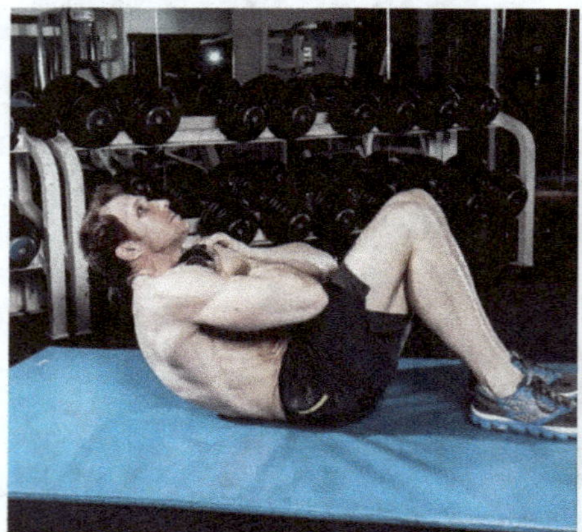

Lie flat on the floor holding a dumbbell to your chest with both hands. Contract your abs to lift your upper back off the floor and curl your chest to your knees. Pause, and then lower.

3 B LOW RUSSIAN TWIST

SETS 3 **REPS** 12 each side **TEMPO** 2010 **REST** 45sec

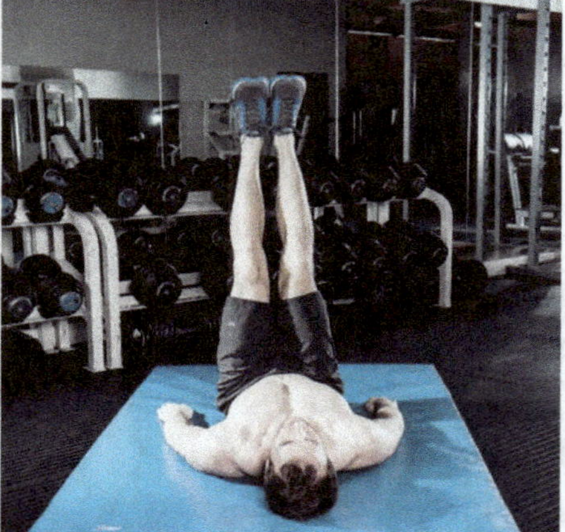

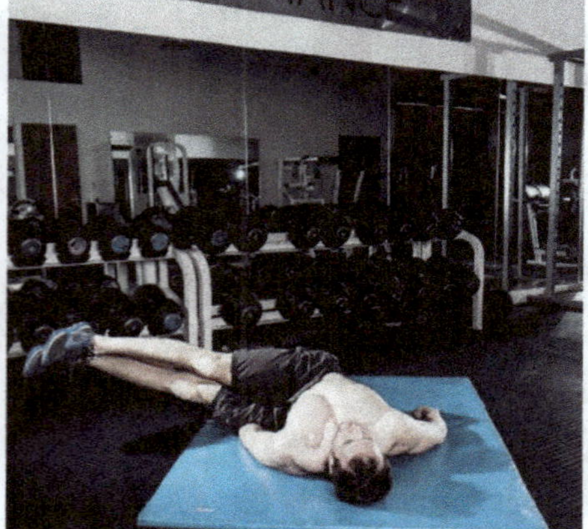

Lie with your back flat on the floor and bring your legs to one side and then the other, like a set of windscreen wipers. Do the movement slow and under control.

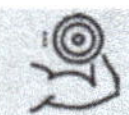

WEEK 4

It's the final week, so give it everything you've got

WORKOUT 1 **CHEST AND BACK**

EXERCISE	SETS	REPS	TEMPO	REST
1A Incline bench press	5	8	2010	10SEC
1B Wide-grip seated row	5	8	2111	45SEC
2A Lying dumbbell pull-over	4	10	2010	10SEC
2B Lying dumbbell flye	4	10	2010	45SEC
3A Wide-grip lat pull-down	3	12	2111	10SEC
3B Cable cross-over	3	12	2111	45SEC

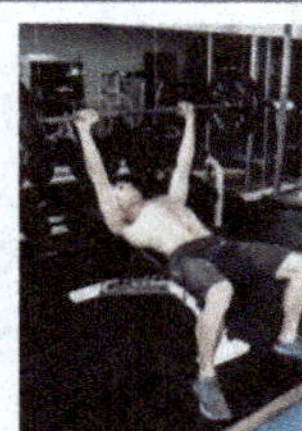

WORKOUT 2 **LEGS AND CORE**

EXERCISE	SETS	REPS	TEMPO	REST
1A Deadlift	5	8	1010	10SEC
1B Squat	5	8	2010	45SEC
2A Leg extension	4	10	1110	10SEC
2B Leg curl	4	10	1110	45SEC
3A Bicycle	3	12	1111	10SEC
3B Oblique crunch	3	12 EACH SIDE	1111	45SEC

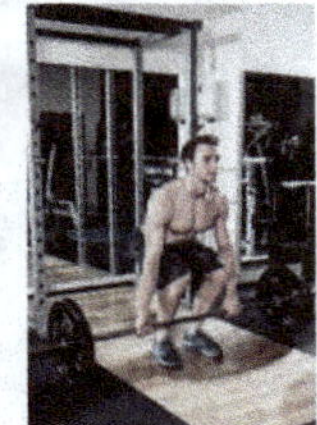

WORKOUT 3 **BICEPS AND TRICEPS**

EXERCISE	SETS	REPS	TEMPO	REST
1A Weighted chin-up	5	8	2010	10SEC
1B Weighted triceps dip	5	8	2110	45SEC
2A EZ-bar preacher curl	4	10	2111	10SEC
2B Lying EZ-bar extension	4	10	2010	45SEC
3A Spider curl	3	12	2110	10SEC
3B Cable rope overhead triceps extension	3	12	2010	45SEC

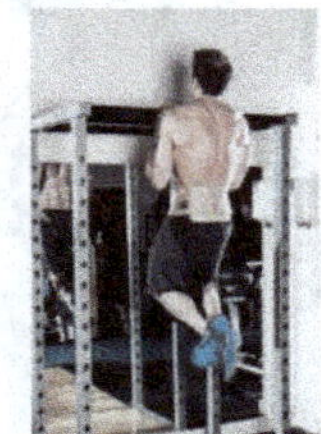

WORKOUT 4 **SHOULDERS AND CORE**

EXERCISE	SETS	REPS	TEMPO	REST
1A Push press	5	8	20X0	10SEC
1B EZ-bar upright row	5	8	2110	45SEC
2A Cable lateral raise	4	10	2110	10SEC
2B Cable face pull	4	10	2110	45SEC
3A Weighted crunch	3	12	1110	10SEC
3B Lower-body Russian twist	3	12 EACH SIDE	1110	45SEC

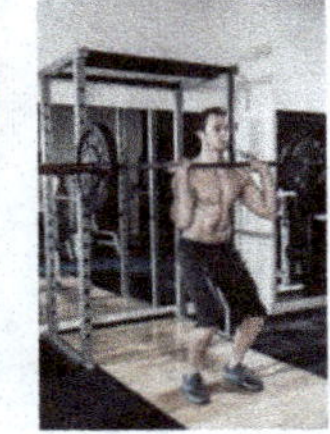

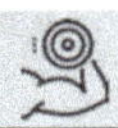

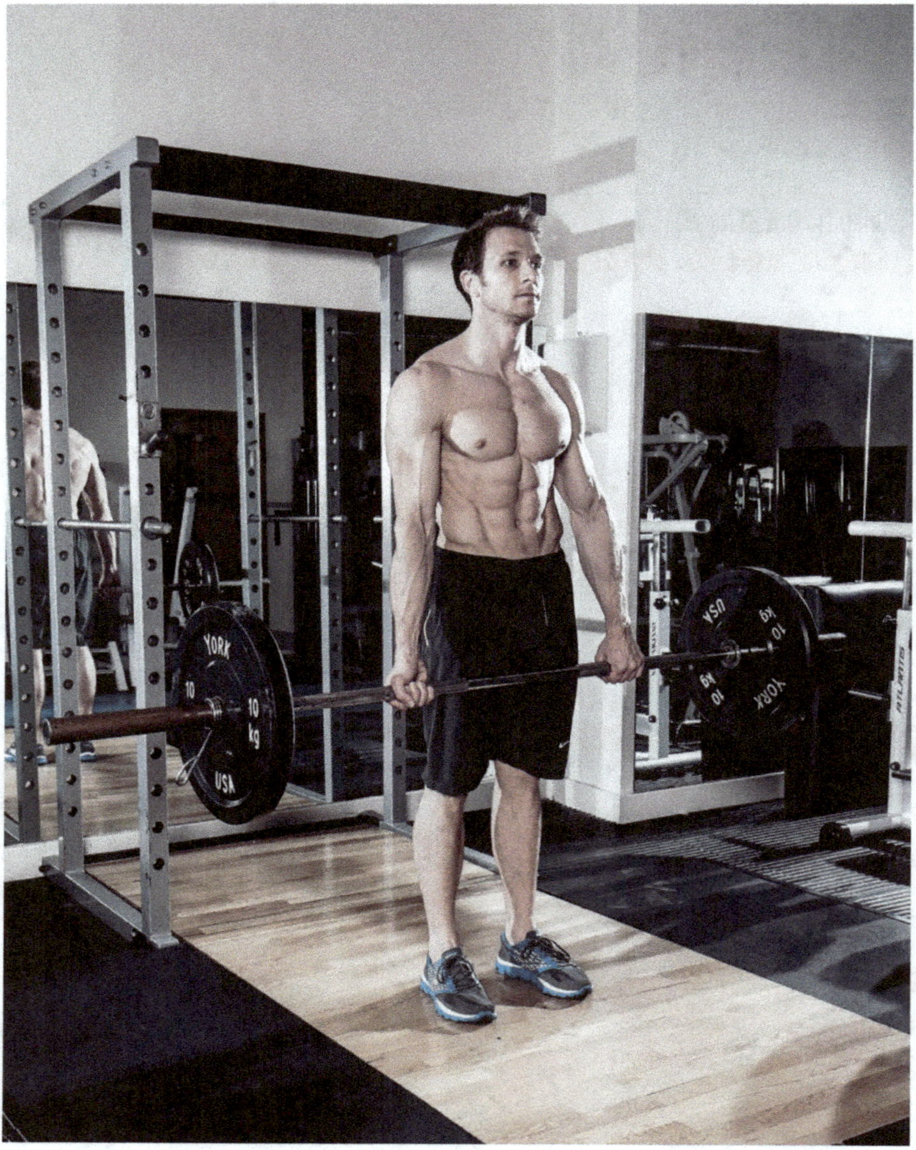